RETAINING
THE MIND

RETAINING THE MIND

How the Foods We Eat Affect Our Brain

William E. Walsh, MD, FACA

MCP Books, Maitland

MCP Books
2301 Lucien Way #415
Maitland, FL 32751
407.339.4217
www.MCPBooks.com

ISBN-13: 978-1-63413-980-9
LCCN: 2016917096

Distributed by Itasca Books

Cover Design by Alan Pranke
Typeset by Alexis Cooke

Printed in the United States of America

Other Books by Dr. Walsh

Home Allergies: Don't Let Your Home Make You Sick

Food Allergies: The Complete Guide to
Understanding and Relieving Your Food Allergies

The Food Allergy Book: The Foods that Cause You
Pain and Discomfort and How to Take Them out of
Your Diet

Treating Food Allergy, My Way!: Exploring the Most
Important Food Allergies, Second Edition

Treating Sinus, Migraine, and Cluster Headaches,
My Way!: An Allergist's Approach to Headache
Treatment

Treating Food Allergy, My Way!: Exploring the Most
Important Food Allergies

Contents

Acknowledgments

Many people helped prepare this book and I am deeply grateful. My thanks to the professionals of MCP Books for changing my manuscript into a book: to Kate Ankofski for helping me improve the manuscript; to Ali McManamon for guiding me through the publishing process; to Robin Tinker for helping me reach those who are unfortunate enough to suffer from nerve deterioration; and to Robert Schmidt, editor, for the hours he spent studying and improving my manuscript into the book you hold today.

Thank you to my son, Bill, who helped refine my thoughts while I was writing. His encouragement and that of my family and friends, especially Mary Cecilia and Meredithe, helped me through the many months of committing my experiences to paper. I also thank Molly Behymer of Creative Catering by Molly LLC for her help in devising a diet to guide the reader.

Also essential to this book is the help my staff gave me in caring for my patients. Thank you to all of you. I appreciate the kindness and competence of Dr. Bill Hicks in accepting responsibility for my patients when I retired and for the wonderful foreword he has provided. His words once again remind me of how much I miss my patients, who also became my friends.

And last, and of supreme importance, thanks to my wonderful patients who guided me on my path of understanding how our modern diet impacts the brain. Without your help, I could not continue to work to solve the mystery of how our diet damages our brain and kills our nerves.

Foreword

I first met Dr. Bill Walsh and his wife, Cec, in 2010. I had just completed my Allergy and Immunology fellowship and was ready to start a new career. Dr. Walsh was ready to retire after 40 years in private allergy practice in Saint Paul, Minnesota, and I was hoping to step in as the new allergist. The first thing that was evident to me upon walking through the doors of Dr. Walsh's practice was that his patients adored him. They felt listened to, cared for, and validated. His would not be an easy act to follow.

I had the honor of working beside Dr. Walsh in the six months before his retirement. Six years later, I happily call him a friend. Knowing what I do now, I understand why his patients love him so much. Dr. Walsh's motivation in practicing medicine was never prestige, or money, or notoriety. It was—and remains—the desire to help people. I do my best to bring to my practice the sincere goodwill that his patients have come to expect, though I am no Dr. Walsh. It's been over five years since he retired and his patients still ask about him on a regular basis. So often I hear: "What's Dr. Walsh up to?" or "I was miserable until I met Dr. Walsh," and even "Dr. Walsh was lifesaving."

In short, he is sorely missed by many.

It is not just Dr. Walsh's sincerity that makes him special; it is also his unique medical perspective. He happens to be an allergist whose diet has affected his own health for many years. His personal experience informs the way he thinks about health—his own and others. In this book, he discusses how his views are not always perfectly aligned with what he refers to as "evidence-based medicine," but how they have been profoundly helpful for himself and others, nonetheless.

Perhaps the most special thing that Dr. Walsh does—which is rare not just among doctors but among people everywhere—is truly listen. I don't mean the kind of polite listening with excellent eye contact and nodding at the correct times; I'm talking about listening to hear and listening to learn. His mantra, which I understood within an hour of meeting him, is: Always listen to the patient. It takes a unique and rare blend of humility and self-confidence to sit across from a patient as if you are a pupil. This is something that I've learned from Dr. Walsh that isn't taught well in medical school. Dr. Walsh takes what he learns from his teachers—his patients—and forms patterns and insights.

As you read this book you will find multiple references to patients whom Dr. Walsh has followed. Many of them may well be those who are in my office today asking about his well-being. Their health improved under his care and, in addition, they felt regarded. It's easy to see from Retaining the Mind that Dr. Walsh's interactions have altered his understanding and resulted in rethinking his medical beliefs. So often as doctors we try to fit a patient into the confines of what we have been taught. Dr. Walsh is mindful of those confines, but continues to be willing to explore outside of them.

Now, after retiring from a successful medical practice, instead of going to the beach, he is driven to share this knowledge in order to help others. He combines his personal experience of food sensitivities with years of listening to thousands of patients to bring you the recommendations in this book.

Much of what is included in this book is not pulled from medical textbooks or journals; rather it is from a doctor who has always been open to learning from his patients. His knowledge and careful attention have afforded him a unique perspective that is new and different. Now he wants to pass this to you.

William Brent Hicks, MD

Board certified in allergy and immunology

Member, American College of Allergy, Asthma, and Immunology

Introduction

How I Suffered Early Alzheimer's Disease and Recovered from It

While working as a consultant allergist, I evaluated and treated hundreds of new patients each year, referred to me by their primary medical caregivers because they suffered illnesses caused by the environment or diet. However, until I retired, I did not realize that I was being stalked by the illness that I dreaded most: nerve deterioration that was destroying my ability to talk and think.

This deterioration of the nerves takes on many forms, including mild cognitive impairment, Parkinson's disease, Huntington's disease (formerly called Huntington's chorea), stroke, multiple sclerosis, amyotrophic lateral sclerosis, diabetic neuropathy, and others—as well as Alzheimer's disease.

I first realized that I was suffering mental deterioration while I was introducing a speaker at a luncheon—a four-minute introduction that should have been easy. It was a disaster.

In the weeks before the luncheon I suspected I was in trouble. As I practiced presenting the introduction I found I could not remember the words of the simple, short speech. When I found that I was unable to give the introduction without notes, I tried to memorize it. I couldn't memorize it. I came to the conclusion that I had to write it down and read it to the luncheon guests. When the time came for me to give the introduction, even though I was reading it, I still missed parts of what I meant to say and the parts I got out of my mouth were accompanied by lots of "ohs" and "ahs." I suspect that the audience did not know what I was saying, and to this day I shudder when I think of that speech!

I should have been able to give that introduction easily. I had treated patients for forty years before my retirement. In my consulting practice, I had been seeing patients referred by other doctors, sending these patients back to their doctors when I finished treating them, and continually evaluating and treating new patients. To maintain this practice I needed hundreds of new patients each year and one of the major means of recruiting them was to give talks to referring doctors and to the general public, often at conferences. I had given many hour-long speeches with ease, and knew that I shouldn't have stumbled over a four-minute introduction.

But I did. I stumbled because intact memory is essential for a presentation by a speaker presenting without notes. The speaker must time the speech to fit into the allotted time, organize the speech into successive steps, implant these steps in his mind, and change the tenor of the talk depending on the audience's reactions. During the speech he must mentally check through each successive step, speak the sentence he is currently presenting, and prepare the next sentence for presentation, while all the time retaining control of his body posture and gestures. Speaking before an audience is easy if the speaker is experienced; it can be impossible if an experienced speaker suffers mental deterioration.

I realized, as I found myself stumbling through the speech, that I was losing control of my thinking.

Further indicating that my mental ability was deteriorating, in ordinary conversation I was having more and more trouble forming sentences. I realized that I was in the early stages of mental deterioration similar to the deterioration recorded in cases of Alzheimer's disease. I became convinced—and still am convinced—that I was suffering the effects of this disease (or one which shares its symptoms). (It should be noted that Alzheimer's disease, at this time, can only be confirmed via autopsy. As I am not yet to that stage of my life, I am forced to use my decades of experience in the medical field to make this self-diagnosis.)

From my experience as an allergist, I had learned that I needed to avoid certain foods and beverages because they seriously interfere with my sleep. I knew that avoiding them would help me to sleep soundly at night, and I suspected that they were also a major cause of the nerve deterioration symptoms I was experiencing. I further realized that I needed to compulsively follow the advice I had given to so many patients: I needed to avoid all the foods that I knew caused my patients to experience the symptoms of nerve damage.

I began to compulsively follow the diet I had developed and used for years to prevent my patients' migraine headaches—and the results have been highly gratifying. The distressing symptoms of mental deterioration have subsided strikingly. I am again able to give a speech or present at a conference. I can formulate complete sentences in ordinary conversation.

On the other hand, if I return to eating the offending foods, in ordinary conversation I again form sentences poorly. The stumbling sentences continue to affect me for about twenty-four hours after I scurry back onto my diet, eliminating the foods that hinder my conversation.

I hope my story helps you to understand the following principles:

- Avoiding certain foods can reverse the many conditions caused by nerve damage—including damage to the nerves of the brain.
- The nerves of the brain can recover from years of abuse.
- If I can do it, you can learn how to do it, as well.

That idea that you can reverse mental deterioration—and other conditions of nerve damage—is the first reason I decided to write this book. A second reason soon followed.

A conversation in a restaurant prompted me to return to writing about illnesses caused by our modern diet. Actually, I did not need much prompting because watching the words flow from my mind, onto paper—carrying thoughts that can help people feel well—fascinates me. (And, after years of treating patients, I have much to tell you.) I especially want to concentrate on a common and poorly understood human misery that has always fascinated me: food sensitivity—especially the sensitivity to certain food chemicals we use in our modern diet.

I will use my years of experience and knowledge of the reactions we can have to foods to help you understand food sensitivity, because food sensitivity affects many, many people. In fact, if you even suspect you are sensitive to foods, you probably are. Food sensitivity truly is that common.

As I was saying earlier, one night I was enjoying a pleasant meal in a restaurant with my friends Mickey and Peter. During our conversation, Mickey asked me what aspect of working with my patients I enjoyed the most. I told her that I enjoyed treating patients who suffered from reactions after eating food. You see, in my practice, I evaluated and treated thousands of patients with food sensitivity. I treated so many that, within the first few minutes of listening to their symptoms, I could usually tell why my patients were suffering—and the foods that were causing the suffering.

Mickey was surprised at my response and replied, "I thought that food allergy was very difficult to diagnose and treat."

"It can be," I replied. "But if you know certain information you will understand why many people suffer from eating specific foods."

A Short Introduction to a Confusing Problem
Using that as my starting point, I told her that, during my first years of medical practice, I did not understand why foods make people

suffer—or what foods were responsible. My training should have told me why people suffer from food allergies. After all, I had been a fellow of the Mayo Clinic's program in allergy and immunology—an excellent program in an excellent institution. I had passed the tests of the American Board of Allergy and Immunology that certified that I was an allergy specialist. In spite of all this preparation, I still did not know why patients were suffering symptoms they attributed to their diets. I thought these patients must be wrong; food could not be causing their symptoms—wasn't it innocent of the charges?

After years of studying food sensitivity in my patients, however, I discovered they were right. In doubting them, I had been wrong. They had much to teach me.

What My Patients Taught Me

Over the years, my patients told me about foods that caused distressing symptoms like frequent headaches, recurrent diarrhea, persistent constipation, dreadful itching, and many other chronic, miserable symptoms. As I evaluated and treated these patients, I realized that they were suffering from sensitivity to certain foods. Patients I treated taught me more and more until I finally better understood what was causing them to suffer.

I was so grateful for this knowledge that I resolved to pass this information on to my patients, to their primary doctors, and even to people who would never come to me for evaluation. With that as my goal, I eventually published four books on people's reactions to their diets. Even after I made available this information about the symptoms caused by eating certain foods, people who suffered from such symptoms still came to me for help.

Unfortunately, for most people, the identity of the foods that cause them so much distress is unknown. How can you avoid the harm they cause if you do not know which foods to avoid—or you simply do not know their dangers? You need this first layer of knowledge to help you avoid these foods and end their ability to harm you.

As I talked to my friends in that restaurant and realized how little the general public knew about how foods could harm them, I knew I needed to write again about food sensitivity.

My Final Reason for Writing This Book

The third reason for writing this book is that, frankly, retirement has given me more time to think about the lessons my patients taught me. During my years in practice I was so busy that I had little time to think deeply about the knowledge I had gained. I did not fully appreciate the grave harm caused by years of eating our modern diet.

After some thought, I realized that if I could point out the foods you should avoid, and the reasons for avoiding them, you (and everyone you know) could begin to relieve the symptoms that plague you. And, of course, even if you are free of symptoms at this time, it's important to learn about the possibility of this situation occurring as soon as possible in case, in the future, foods bring you your own distressing problems.

A dear friend best expressed, in a few words, the aim of this book. When she reflected on my recovery from Alzheimer symptoms she stated: "You came back to life." She was right. For me, losing the ability to think, talk, and feed and cloth myself would be the same as dying. If you (or someone you know) suffer these symptoms, I want to bring you back to life.

PART 1

Theory, Science, and Conclusions

Chapter 1
The Foods That Make Us Sick

At the most basic level, foods cause illnesses because they contain significant amounts of certain chemicals. It is the chemicals in foods that make us sick, not the foods themselves. These chemicals are:

1. Monosodium glutamate (abbreviated as MSG)
2. Low-calorie sweeteners
3. Gluten
4. Refined sugar
5. Citric acid
6. Lactose

You may already be familiar with the harm attributed to gluten and refined sugar. As you look at the rest of the list, you may ask yourself "Can these other food chemicals also cause problems?" My answer is: "Yes, in my experience, all of these food chemicals can cause symptoms in sensitive people."

If sensitive people could remove the above chemicals from their food; for instance, the citric acid from oranges or the monosodium glutamate from cheese, these foods would lose their power to cause harm. Sensitive eaters could eat the foods and feel well. I'm happy to say that the avoidance does not have to be complete, because even people who are sensitive to these chemicals can tolerate them in small amounts. Therefore, sensitive sufferers can avoid their potential for harm by limiting their consumption to whatever amount they can tolerate.

If you share a sensitivity to one (or all) of these food chemicals, this book will help you identify the foods that contain excesses of these chemicals so you can avoid causing yourself distress.

Our modern diet contains high levels of these chemicals, however, and they entered our diet only recently. They were not part of the diet of our ancestors countless centuries ago when our genes were being formed; our ancestors did not produce and eat these food chemicals until relatively recent times, a very short period in our evolutionary history. In the many millions of years of evolution that programmed our genes to tolerate some food chemicals and avoid others, a few thousand years is only a blink of the eye. In short, our bodies were not genetically prepared for our current diet.

A List of Principles Guiding Our Study of Food Sensitivity

Now that you are aware of the suspect food chemicals, let us look at the principles that have guided me in my study of food sensitivities:

- The foods themselves do not cause reactions; the chemicals they contain cause the reactions.
- From an evolutionary viewpoint, the high levels of chemicals are recent additions to our diets.
- With their recent addition to our diets, many of us have not developed the genetic ability to fully tolerate and metabolize these foods.
- Usually we tolerate these food chemicals well in our early years but then lose this tolerance as we age.
- Not everyone shares this genetic susceptibility; many people tolerate these chemicals throughout life.
- Most of the chemical-containing foods are otherwise good foods.
- These six diet chemicals, because they are made up of small molecules, cannot cause allergic reactions. (Allergy-causing

molecules are larger.)

- ✻ Because they do not cause the symptoms of allergic reactions, these chemicals seldom precipitate symptoms of allergy such as hay fever–like sneezing or dangerous anaphylaxis.
- ✻ Symptoms caused by reactions to these food chemicals usually appear hours to days after eating the foods, not within minutes of eating them. (Reactions to food allergies typically strike as the food is eaten or soon after.)
- ✻ Food allergies can be triggered by minute amounts of food, but reactions caused by food sensitivities require eating larger quantities.

There are exceptions to these characteristics (for instance, we may find an occasional baby who suffers from a food sensitivity) but these exceptions are infrequent.

In this list of relationships, you should realize that there is one important concept: We are discussing food sensitivity, not a food allergy. This is an important distinction because the causes of food allergies and food sensitivities differ—and an allergy is far easier to diagnose. They also act differently: a food allergy is the arrow that strikes suddenly; a food sensitivity is the sluggishly moving catapult that slowly pounds the city wall.

Back to the Restaurant Conversation

Now that you have some feeling for what it means to have a sensitivity to food chemicals, let's return to the restaurant and the conversation with Mickey and Peter I told you about earlier. I had mentioned to them that the differences between food allergies and food sensitivities confuse many people, but that understanding this distinction is essential to understanding why foods cause distress.

I went on to explain that the most common cause of suffering related to food intake is not an allergy to foods. It is, instead, a food sensitivity—the inability to tolerate certain foods that are common in our diet.

I regret that many unfortunate people suffer because they eat foods that contain these food chemicals, which are well tolerated by many other people. After all, a few of these foods are known to be good for us, and—if we can tolerate them—should be included in our diets.

Naming This Food Sensitivity

I find it difficult to think of food sensitivity as a "disease" or an "illness." To me, naming it a disease implies an infectious or cancerous cause. Calling it an illness or sickness implies much the same. I believe that the sensitivity to these food chemicals is not an illness, disease, or sickness. Instead, it is a normal result of aging, similar to other conditions that accompany aging (including baldness or decreased muscle tone). Calling these latter conditions illnesses, infections, or cancer just doesn't sound right, does it? However, I must use these terms to discuss food sensitivities in this book because I know of no better terms to use.

If some day we can reverse aging, maybe we can then reverse food sensitivities, but until that day I believe we are forced to use the terms sensitivity or intolerance because that is what this situation is: an increased sensitivity to—or intolerance of—certain food chemicals because our aging digestive systems cannot handle high levels of the chemicals.

To avoid naming all six food chemicals each time I discuss them as a group, I will refer to them as the "aging chemicals." As we examine any one of the six individual food chemicals I will use the name of that chemical followed by either "sensitivity" or "intolerance" (for example, "citric acid sensitivity" or "citric acid intolerance").

The majority of people who suffer from the food sensitivity we will be discussing do so because they are growing older. Sensitivity to this group of food chemicals not only accompanies aging but also causes a number of the discomforts and disabilities we associate with growing older through their effect on our nerves. Nerves participate in the control of our muscles, organs, hormones, and every other area of our body—including the brain. So, when these chemicals impact the nerves in our brains and bodies, the results can be: diminished thinking capacity; fading memory; sensation loss that weakens our balance and degrades our toilet habits; and the lessening of the emotional/physical coordination that leads to intimacy.

When we consider these diet chemicals' profound effects on our life and behavior as we age, we realize that there is truly no better name for them than the aging chemicals.

Caution:

Although I will be presenting a lot of medically based information in this book, this book is not intended to diagnose your condition—so do not try to make it your doctor. When I was in practice, I could not diagnose my patients' illnesses unless I saw them, examined them, and studied the results of any necessary tests. This book cannot see you, examine you, or arrange for tests. Instead, its purpose is to acquaint you with common and harmful conditions that arise from the modern diet and to prompt you to discuss with your caregiver the possibility that you are similarly affected by sensitivity to certain foods.

If you suffer from any diagnosed food allergies you must continue to limit or avoid the foods that cause your allergic symptoms while also avoiding the aging chemicals. If you suffer from combined food allergy and food sensitivity, your food avoidance will be more complicated and the help of a dietician may be essential to make sure you continue eating a healthy diet.

Chapter 2

Why the Effect of the Aging Chemicals Hides So Successfully

The Effect of the Aging Chemicals Hides from the Sufferer

Food sensitivity hides from the affected person for two main reasons.

The First Reason

First, affected people typically believe that foods that they have tolerated without symptoms in the past cannot cause their headaches or abdominal distress today. However, this idea is wrong. My patients' stories showed me that foods which were tolerated well earlier in life can cause miserable symptoms with age. Not only does this happen, but it happens frequently. This later-in-life sensitivity becomes easier to believe when sufferers realize that, as aging brings many changes (including, as we've discussed, baldness and decreased muscle tone), for them it also brings a lower tolerance to many food chemicals.

Not everybody loses hair or muscle tone, just as not everybody loses tolerance to these aging chemicals. But if they do lose this tolerance, they must avoid excessive eating of the offending foods—eating no more than they can tolerate—or they will suffer.

The Second Reason

The second reason affected people fail to recognize the dietary source of their distress is that they can eat limited amounts of these same chemicals without experiencing symptoms. Often my patients

9

asked me: "But I just ate (or drank) some of it yesterday and had no trouble. Why should it trouble me today?"

My answer: "Yesterday you did not eat (or drink) enough to trigger your stomach pain and diarrhea (or headaches) but today you exceeded the amount that you can tolerate and now you are suffering. It takes the body about three days to eliminate the gluten (or whatever the offending chemical was) that you ate, so over-indulgence over those three days can accumulate sufficient food chemicals in your body to trigger symptoms. Once you are suffering symptoms, this same one-to-three days must pass before you can safely return to eating limited amounts of that food."

People suffering from ingesting the aging chemicals need only realize that, although as youngsters they were able to eat lots of certain foods without symptoms, now that they are older they can no longer tolerate the same quantities of these foods. Further, they must realize that eating small amounts of these foods without symptoms does not mean that they can eat larger amounts without suffering. Once they comprehend these two factors, this sensitivity can no longer hide from them.

If you understand this, then the troubles caused by the aging chemicals can no longer hide from you.

The Effect of These Chemicals Hides from Doctors

Not only does the impact of these sensitivities hide from sensitive people, it also hides from doctors, again for two reasons.

The First Reason

First, no test can diagnose food sensitivity. For instance, there is a test for celiac disease but in this book I am not discussing celiac disease, even though I will be discussing a sensitivity to gluten. (If you have celiac disease, this is not the book for you—you must follow the treatment for celiac disease, not the treatment that I advocate here.) In the years I spent in my allergy practice I diagnosed and treated hundreds of gluten-sensitive patients and took many, many tests for celiac disease; only three of my patients had the positive tests that diagnose celiac disease. All the rest had sensitivity to the aging chemicals that we are discussing here.

Although celiac disease is relatively rare, food sensitivity is common. I treated hundreds of food-sensitive patients. Those hundreds of patients, although impressive, are only a tiny fraction of the millions of people suffering from food sensitivities.

The Second Reason

The second reason the symptoms caused by these aging chemicals are able to hide from doctors can be summed up in two terms: "evidence-based medicine" and "medical peer review." "Evidence-based medicine" means that a reputable doctor should provide evidence— by using appropriate tests—that a patient suffers an identified disease or sickness and can follow the treatment that clinical trials show is most effective and least harmful. "Medical peer review" means that the clinical trials on which your doctor bases her treatment must be judged to be competent and reliable by experts in the condition being studied.

A doctor treating a patient affected by the aging chemicals has almost no peer-reviewed clinical trials to depend on (except in a few instances that we will discuss later). The reason she does not have these treatment trials to depend on is that the trials need a group of patients proven—through recognized laboratory tests or x-ray tests—to suffer the sickness or illness being studied. Unfortunately, in the majority of cases, a food chemical sensitivity cannot be diagnosed because no tests exist that can diagnose it. Therefore, doctors have little or no "peer-reviewed," "evidence-based" treatment to follow.

An example of the same frustrating lack of evidence-based

treatment exists for the millions of people who suffer the ill-defined pain called "headaches." The pain itself is difficult to define; there are many causes of headaches, and many of these causes cannot be identified. As in food sensitivity, because doctors cannot diagnose the cause of the headaches, peer-reviewed, evidence-based approaches to the treatment of some headaches are not available.

Of course, as with headaches, this lack of confirmatory testing does not mean that these chemicals cause no pain or suffering—or that they plague only a few. In fact, millions suffer pain and distress from these chemicals.

So what should the doctor do in a situation where a patient is suffering, the cause cannot be diagnosed by tests, and the symptoms are non-specific? I know no satisfactory answer to that question. As you pity the patient, also pity the doctor; she does not know what to do for her patients who suffer from these sensitivities.

What Happens Since This Food Sensitivity Cannot Be Diagnosed by Medical Tests

There is one more consequence to the aging chemicals' ability to hide from doctors: I am seriously hampered in telling you about the specific causes and outcomes because of our inability to diagnose food sensitivities through medical tests.

It would be different if I were teaching you about a diagnosable illness, like a food allergy that can be identified by skin tests, or asthma that can be identified by pulmonary function tests. In one of those cases, I could tell you the results of clinical trials studying patients with allergies or asthma. Because food sensitivity cannot be confirmed by tests, patients cannot be unequivocally identified, treatment trials cannot be performed, and neither I nor anybody else can provide you with "proven, tested" results.

Even with the lack of evidence-based diagnosis and treatment, you need to know about food chemical sensitivity to determine whether you suffer from it and how to avoid the foods that make you suffer. To help you, I will use the clinical experience I gained during forty years of treating hundreds of sensitive patients.

In the next chapters I will examine each of the six individual aging chemicals: MSG, low-calorie sweeteners, gluten, refined sugar, citric acid, and lactose. I believe we should start our examination of these food chemicals with monosodium glutamate, as it is a potent aging chemical. In fact, to understand the harm caused by all six aging chemicals, you must first understand monosodium glutamate.

Chapter 3
Monosodium Glutamate—the Most Dangerous Food Chemical

The name "monosodium glutamate" signifies an amino acid—glutamic acid (also called glutamate)—accompanied by one ("mono-") sodium ion. Glutamic acid is one of the amino acids that, when tightly bonded to other amino acids, form proteins (including the proteins of our red and white blood cells and muscle). It also forms the protein of organs like the liver, spleen, and brain. Glutamic acid must be part of these proteins. It is essential for life, and it is harmless when tightly bound to, or imprisoned within, protein.

In this chapter we will discuss how breaking apart proteins releases amino acids, including glutamic acid. Once broken free of protein and combined with sodium, glutamic acid floats freely in water, including the water in your bloodstream, and reaches anywhere in your body. In this state, the chemical we will be looking at can be termed "free" glutamic acid, monosodium glutamate, or, simply, MSG.

You need to understand MSG to discover why it is both essential for life and dangerous. Because there is so much information you need to know, I have divided this information into numbered parts:

Part 1: Free Glutamic Acid—a Potent and Worrisome Amino Acid

Part 2: Symptoms Caused by MSG

Part 1:
Free Glutamic Acid—a Potent and Worrisome Amino Acid

There is nothing unusual about amino acids floating freely in the blood stream. Once released from their prisons in proteins, they travel through your body, doing their work of building and repairing the body's proteins—all innocent, all natural, and all helpful. Except, in certain circumstances, when one of these amino acids—glutamic acid—becomes dangerous.

Glutamic acid is dangerous because of its power. When free from its protein prison, glutamic acid serves as a potent neurotransmitter for our nervous system. This means that the nerves use glutamic acid to carry a nerve impulse from one nerve to another (the nerve impulse starts in our brains and ranges throughout our bodies traveling out to the nerves that control our arms, legs, tongues, and everything else). Using glutamic acid as a nerve stimulator solves a huge problem for the nervous system: it helps the brain communicate with the rest of the body.

To understand this process, let's greatly simplify certain situations where your brain stimulates your nerves to trigger actions, from adding up a grocery bill to covering your nose when you sneeze, to running like a gazelle when you see a hungry saber-tooth tiger charging. In all these situations, your brain needs to activate certain nerve cells to count up the bill, cover the sneeze, or run like mad.

Your brain must be very selective in which nerves it stimulates. If every time you are asked to add a grocery bill your nerves prompt you to run full speed through the grocery store bowling over carts and customers, you will be thrown out of the store by the enraged customers. Or if you start covering your sneeze instead of running when charged by a tiger, only the tiger will be happy.

If the nerves that start in your brain and end in your leg muscles delivered only powerful stimulation to your legs' running muscles, never relaxing after this stimulation, your stimulated leg muscles would go into spasm (similar to having an epileptic seizure), preventing you from running, dropping you to the ground, and, again, making the tiger happy.

To prevent this, your brain's command to run away travels through a network of nerves extending from the brain to the nerves that control the leg muscles, the network alternately commanding your leg muscles to extend your leg and then retract it while you run. This network of nerves is like a network of electrical extension cords and has the weakness of these extension cords: short-circuiting if the wires, hot with electricity, touch each other.

To prevent this, extension cords are insulated so the hot wires in an extension cord do not touch the surrounding hot wires and cause uncontrolled, dangerous sparking. Likewise, nerves are insulated from each other with a material called myelin, which prevents them from touching each other and sending bursts of uncontrolled nerve impulses careening through your convulsing body.

So, if nerves are completely insulated from each other, how does a stimulus pass through the nerve network? To pass stimulation down the net of nerves, a chemical leaps across the spaces between nerves (the nerve synapses), from the nerves that are stimulated to the nerves which need to be stimulated. This chemical stimulates the next nerves in the network, which then stimulate the next, until the nerves that extend or retract the leg muscles are reached. By alternatively extending and then retracting your leg muscle, your body moves, allowing you to flee from the tiger.

To activate these nerves—to flee the tiger—this chemical acts much like a spray of rocket fuel, allowing stimulated nerves to pass on the stimulus to run. It must force the receiving nerve to obey. Unfortunately, a chemical so harsh—so commanding—might damage or even kill the receiving nerves.

18

The most common chemical used by the body to stimulate nerves is the neurostimulating amino acid glutamic acid—MSG. Its action is very powerful, but can also be very dangerous to nerves if it is not rapidly cleared away from the space between the nerves before it harms the nerve.

Once the glutamic acid is cleared from the space between two nerves, the first nerve relaxes and stops stimulating the next nerve. If this nerve is stimulating a muscle that makes the leg extend, ending the stimulus allows the extending muscle to relax while another nerve activates the muscle that contracts the leg. This quick extension/contraction powers the running that helps evade the tiger.

When Glutamic Acid Causes Harm

Unfortunately, the "washing out" of the MSG from the synapse may—and in many people does—weaken as we age. The weakness turns MSG from helpful to harmful and from neurostimulant to neurotoxin. (I am using the terms "toxic" and "toxin" to indicate a poison that is produced naturally by living things. A substance which is toxic can vary from mild and hardly noticeable to deadly.) Once the MSG becomes toxic, then arise the punishing symptoms suffered by people sensitive to the glutamic acid of MSG.

In brain injury or disease, the mechanism that removes the glutamic acid released in nerve stimulation can fail. This allows excess glutamic acid to accumulate around the nerve cells, causing such injury to the nerves that large numbers of calcium ions enter the nerve cell, bulging out the cell, and harming or even killing it. Many doctors and scientists believe that this is one of the processes that damage the brain in stroke, amyotrophic lateral sclerosis, and Alzheimer's disease. It may also be a cause of epileptic seizures.

In short, glutamic acid, MSG, is dangerous.

A Note of Explanation:

Before continuing our discussion about MSG I want to acknowledge that the companies that produce the food flavoring, MSG, probably believe it causes no harm. I also acknowledge that it is a natural and effective flavor enhancer. The FDA considers the addition of MSG to foods to be "generally recognized as safe," but I am sorry that I cannot agree. It is not safe for those sensitive to the nerve damage inflicted by MSG.

Why All This Discussion about This Amino Acid?

Obviously, MSG plays an essential role in keeping us alive—without it, our nerves would communicate only poorly, and our ancestors would have been fine feasts for tigers, lions, and other predators.

However, in many people the good that MSG does becomes overshadowed by the harm it causes. As you learn that MSG is essential to life, you must also learn that it is dangerous. MSG sensitivity explains why so many people living in our modern society suffer such a sad multitude of painful and disabling illnesses.

I am a specialist in both food allergy and food sensitivity. I am not a specialist in neurology—nor do I want to portray myself as a specialist in that field. However, I had to venture into the field of neurology to tell you about what glutamic acid does. If you understand this information, you will then understand the rest of the discussion about MSG. Applying this knowledge to the other aging chemicals will also help you understand them.

Now let's look at the symptoms that can affect MSG-sensitive people.

Part 2:
Symptoms Caused by MSG

In this section I will use three sources of information to tell you about the symptoms caused by MSG. First, I will tell you about the symptoms I personally experience when I overindulge in food or drink flavored with MSG. Second, I will tell you about the symptoms suffered by a dear friend of mine who first alerted me to the potential harm caused by MSG. Third, I will discuss the ways in which MSG troubled so many of the patients who came to me for evaluation and treatment.

I have already told you that the aging chemicals have affected me for many years. I know my symptoms well; in describing these symptoms to you, I can help you learn about MSG. My symptoms also helped me in evaluating the thousands of patients who came to me for diagnosis and treatment in my allergy specialty practice. Because I shared their symptoms, within a few minutes of visiting with my food-sensitive patients I knew why they suffered—and I could fully sympathize with them.

By the way, even though my patients benefited from my experiences with the aging chemicals—and I was pleased that they did benefit—I would rather not be sensitive to the syndrome. If I knew how to cure it, I would cure myself today and go back to eating a "normal" diet that includes all the fine tasting foods I must avoid.

1) My Symptoms

Sleep disturbance

My most irritating and persistent symptom is sleep disturbance. It comes in two varieties. If I eat a meal with a gross excess of MSG, I simply will not be able to sleep for forty-eight hours. Typically, after two sleepless nights spent looking at my bedroom ceiling, I renew my determination to follow my diet compulsively. That resolution lasts for weeks until another delicious meal full of MSG stares back at me from my plate and my weak willpower tempts me into eating it. This, of course, is followed by another two nights without sleep—and another resolution to avoid the foods.

The next variety of sleep disturbance arises when I eat or drink a slight excess of MSG, much less than the gross excess of the meal that brings the forty-eight-hour sleeplessness. Let me explain what I mean by a "slight excess." As a rule, all of the aging chemicals can be eaten by sensitive people, after all they are all present in acceptable foods and small amounts do not typically cause adverse symptoms. On the other hand, eating or drinking more than these safe amounts can bring uncomfortable symptoms.

Eating a slight excess of MSG affects my sleep, waking me after just four hours feeling tired, forcing me to arise from a sleep that was not refreshing, making me wish I could sleep longer. If I avoid this small excess of MSG for a few days, I return to enjoying a longer and more refreshing sleep. I have found that many of my patients share this four-hour sleep pattern and I feel confident that this pattern is a sign of MSG sensitivity.

More recent—but far more worrisome—symptoms that I have encountered are the memory loss and difficulty speaking I have already described. As MSG interferes with sleep and degrades speech, it also damages memory, which can be horribly worrisome for anyone afflicted by this mental deterioration.

Diarrhea Followed by Constipation

Of lesser distress to me, although not without annoyance, are bouts of diarrhea and constipation that follow eating or drinking excess MSG. Typically, the diarrhea appears hours after a given meal—up to twenty-four hours later—which sets it apart from the quick-appearing diarrhea related to food allergies. The cramping of the diarrhea subsides after several hours, followed by multiple days of constipation that, at times, can be uncomfortable. The whole process lasts for three days after which, if I watch my diet, the bowel movements return to their usual pattern.

I believe that MSG is a major cause of this alternating constipation/diarrhea, and have found that, in sensitive people, reducing the amount of MSG in the diet will return the stool pattern to normal. However, if these sensitive people are unaware that they are sensitive to MSG, and continue to consume MSG, they will continue to suffer an uncomfortable stool pattern. I know that this is so because that is what happened to me before I realized that the source of my chronic constipation arose from my diet—and that it returns when I stray too far from my diet.

Many of my patients sensitive to the aging food chemicals suffer similar bouts of constipation/diarrhea, suggesting that this food sensitivity is a common cause of these symptoms.

Bloating and Weight Gain

I can also tell when my diet makes me bloat. My belt feels tight and forms an uncomfortable band across my waist; I do not feel that uncomfortable tightness if I am avoiding MSG and the other aging chemicals. Further, my bathroom scale goes up by two to five pounds when I consume an excess of these chemicals and goes down by the same amount if avoid them. This weight gain ends with increased urination when I avoid MSG for a few days, pointing to fluid accumulation as the cause of the bloating.

Many food-sensitive patients have told me that they also suffered bloating. You, like me, can also feel it if you suffer this food sensitivity.

We just discussed the sleeplessness, memory loss, difficulty speaking, bloating and constipation/diarrhea caused by MSG. Now let's discuss another common symptom, a very painful symptom, which a friend told me about.

2) My Friend John's Symptoms

John was an artist, a man whose friendship my wife and I treasured for years. We often vacationed together with John and his wife, and he was an art mentor for our young son. Thus, it deeply troubled me when my good friend told me about the severe pain that tormented him. I still remember that day.

John said, "Bill, this past week my cluster headaches returned. They return several times a year and when they return they often stay for several weeks. The pain comes in waves and hurts me so much that at times I bang my head against a wall to try to take my mind away from the pain."

"John, your headaches are that severe?"

"Yes, my recent attack struck about two hours after a meal and I believe that the pain came from a sausage I ate before the pain started."

"Did you find out the ingredients of the sausage?"

"No, but will you call the restaurant and find out the ingredients?"

I agreed to call for a good reason: if I could identify the cause of John's headaches—and if a food caused them—it might give me a clue into how foods cause headaches. I called the restaurant and found that the only suspicious ingredient in the sausage was MSG.

This conversation started my interest in MSG and its relationship to headaches. As long as John avoided MSG, his headaches became fewer and less painful—but they returned when he allowed MSG into his diet.

Cluster Headaches

To give you an idea of the power of MSG in causing severely painful headaches, let's examine these headaches. Cluster headaches strike in a "cluster" of episodes, usually without warning, and usually after weeks or months of being free from headaches. They return daily—sometimes several times in a day—and last anywhere from minutes to hours. They usually bring excruciating pain in or around one eye, but can strike anywhere about the face, neck, and shoulders.

Typically during a cluster headache one eye reddens and tears run from the eye, the skin surrounding the eye swells and reddens, the eyelid droops, and the eye feels like it is being pushed out of its socket. At the same time, the nose stuffs up, the face reddens, sweat blankets the face, and the sufferer moves restlessly. The pain hurts so much that it feels like a hot poker is being stuck in the eye. (No wonder John bangs his head against a wall to distract him from the pain.)

3) My Patients' Symptoms

John's experience prompted me to ask my patients if they suffered headaches and, if they said they did, I asked them to watch their diet to see if MSG causes their headaches.

In my practice, hundreds of new patients consulted me for evaluation and treatment each year, for many years. Many of these patients suffered headaches, they were mostly migraine headaches, with smaller numbers suffering cluster headaches. Through following my advice, many of my patients discovered that the ingestion of MSG preceded their pain. This raises the distinct possibility that in the population at large (not just among my patients), MSG could be bringing tormenting headaches to millions of people.

Part 3:
What Our Symptoms Tell Us about MSG

Example: Cluster Headaches

The stories I related above teach us much about the aging chemicals. John's headaches are typical of cluster headaches: they strongly indicate that stimulation of the trigeminal nerve, the chief sensory nerve of the face, causes the headache pain. This nerve pain refocuses our attention on free glutamic acid (MSG), a major nerve stimulator (neurostimulant) which, when not properly cleared away from the nerve, becomes a nerve toxin (neurotoxin).

This stimulation of the trigeminal nerve, caused by glutamic acid, brings on the severe eye pain that plagues the miserable sufferers of cluster headaches. It also causes the nasal congestion, nasal discharge, eye tearing, and eye redness that accompany cluster headaches. This pain associated with cluster headaches shows that MSG truly stimulates and irritates nerves.

Example: Common Migraine Headaches

My experience with migraine sufferers also tells me (and many other doctors agree) that arteries beneath the scalp cause migraine pain. These headaches, in the form of "common migraine headaches," bring intense, throbbing pain to the head, often accompanied by nausea, vomiting, and extreme sensitivity to light and sound.

Scientists are unsure of the causes of common migraine headaches but the throbbing pain certainly suggests that the pulsating or throbbing of the arteries in the head must be involved. The head has a rich supply of arteries that travel around the head, accompanied intimately by nerves; the intertwining nerves and blood vessels are called "neurovascular bundles" (neuro refers to nerves, while vascular indicates blood vessels). This grouping of

26

nerves and blood vessels occurs not only in the head but also throughout the body.

Nerves control the expansion and constriction of blood vessels; damage to the nerves by MSG may exaggerate this expansion of the arteries of the head, causing swollen blood vessels. Now imagine, in the head, the arteries banging against the damaged nerves they travel with—and you can see why migraine headaches cause a banging, pulsating pain like a swinging door repeatedly closing on a trapped finger. Ouch! Damaged nerves cry for relief; pain is the only cry they can make. The pain of migraine headaches may be our bodies begging us to stop eating MSG.

Examples: Basilar and Familial Hemiplegic Migraines

These two rare forms of migraine headaches also point to the interaction of nerves and arteries in the neurovascular bundles and how this interaction causes migraine headaches. The pain from a basilar migraine comes from an artery in the base of the brain, in the brainstem. An "aura"—a group of sensations such as dizziness, double vision, peculiar odors, and lack of coordination—often alerts the sufferer ten to forty-five minutes before the headache starts. The aura is caused by the inappropriate stimulation of the nerves that control sight, smell, and body coordination and—combined with the pulsating pain of the headache—demonstrate how the arteries and nerves can team up to cause throbbing migraine headaches.

Earlier, I discussed the aging of normal genes and I believe this aging causes common migraine headaches, because aging reduces our ability to clear glutamic acid from around the nerves. In some people the impact of aging may start surprisingly early in life.

Let's turn now to hemiplegic migraines to acknowledge that, at least in certain rare conditions, gene mutation—like aging—can also cause symptoms involving neurotransmitters. Hemiplegic migraines can be confused with basilar migraines because the symptoms of the two are generally the same except that muscle weakness accompanies the attacks of hemiplegic migraine.

The value of putting hemiplegic migraines under our magnifying glass is that the cause of this type of migraine headache is known—and it is genetic. Mutations in specific genes (CACNA1A, ATP1A2, SCN1A, and PRRT2) cause it. Therefore, as I mentioned, in addition to aging, gene mutation can cause migraine headaches.

Scientists have discovered the function of these mutant genes in hemiplegic migraine and it shifts our attention back to glutamic acid. These mutated genes provide instructions for making proteins that help neurotransmitters pass their stimulation to the next nerve. (Remember that the leading neurotransmitter in the brain is glutamic acid/MSG.) Because of these mutated genes, the body only poorly flushes MSG from around nerves, making the possessor of the genes especially sensitive to the harmful effects of MSG and especially susceptible to migraine headaches.

Perhaps, in aging people, similar gene mutations—present since birth and waiting to be triggered—predispose them to these headaches. If so, these mutations hide well because researchers studying aging people still seek them. If they are present, and researchers could find them, these researchers would finally possess the diagnostic tests they desire to perform the peer-reviewed clinical tests that would better identify the cause of the headaches. That would be wonderful.

In the meantime, we can apply what we have learned from basilar and hemiplegic migraines about MSG-damaged nerves causing headaches to understanding their participation in causing symptoms other than headaches. The chronic symptoms of diarrhea and constipation that trouble so many people, including me, can obviously be caused by MSG irritation of the nerves in the neurovascular bundles in the intestine.

Poor sleep is another condition explained by MSG-irritated nerves. Areas that control sleep/wakefulness run through the brain, from the spinal cord to the cerebral cortex (in other words, from the bottom to the top of the brain). The sleeplessness that occurs after excess MSG eating—and the four-hour broken sleep pattern resulting from continuous MSG eating—must be caused by this irritation of brain nerve cells in these wake/sleep areas of the brain, in people who poorly handle large dietary loads of MSG.

There may be those who object to these conclusions, who claim that MSG cannot affect the brain. Let them call me at two o'clock in the morning after an MSG meal while I lie awake, looking at the ceiling, and I will tell them what I think of their objections.

Part 4:
Why Avoiding MSG Is So Important for Any Person Desiring to Avoid the Aging It Causes

So far in our discussion of MSG I have been giving you enough information to realize that, if you are sensitive to MSG (glutamic acid), you should consume less of it. To do this you must avoid many foods and beverages you enjoy. Your reward for this avoidance is a resurrection to health of the nerves it has been damaging.

One example of your reward is a return to restful sleep. Many scientific studies show that a lack of restful sleep is destructive to the health of the body and hastens mental decline. In other words: poor sleep ages your brain—and your body.

I dread aging; I hate losing my freedom, and do not want to start depending on the care of others, or to need help even in my toilet care. I want to continue to enjoy the white of the winter snow, the planting and growing of flowers, and the writing of books. The fear of accelerated aging scared me so much that, when I found myself sinking into mental deterioration, I resolved to change my diet because I knew that it was the only way to avoid these humiliating consequences.

If you also want to live independently, to enjoy the beauty of nature, and to not need to live in a memory unit, you must be careful of your diet. With care we all have a great chance to maintain the independence and self-respect that you and I so desperately desire.

If MSG Is So Bad, Why Is It So Widely Used in Our Diet?

MSG stimulates nerves; among the nerves it stimulates are the nerves in the taste buds on the surface of the mouth, tongue, and throat. This stimulation does not confer a particular flavor on foods but it accentuates the flavor of any food with which it is combined. This pleasing sensation makes almost any food taste great. I can usually tell when a food or drink contains high levels of MSG because the taste is exquisite. This excellence of taste warns me that imminent poor sleep, uncomfortable abdominal distress, and slowing of the brain will make me regret eating it. Most of the time I do not eat beyond the first taste because my willpower wins. Unfortunately, as I mentioned, sometimes my willpower sleeps (and I don't).

Part 5:
Identifying the Sources of MSG
Plants Altered by Farmers to Have High Levels of Free Glutamic Acid

As I've mentioned, foods which have been altered to contain higher levels of free glutamic acid taste much better than foods from original, unaltered plants, which have lower levels of this amino acid. Over many centuries, farmers picked out the better-tasting foods to replant, steadily improving the food's taste, while also increasing its content of the free MSG that confers the improved taste. In the present day, many of our "natural" foods are actually highly modified from the way they originally appeared, are no longer in their truly natural forms, and contain increased levels of MSG.

MSG-sensitive people can eat these "natural" foods but must do so with some caution, eating and drinking only as much of these MSG-containing foods and beverages as they can tolerate. A list of these foods is below:

Corn

Known in much of the world as "maize," its original form seems to have been a grass-like plant domesticated (meaning that it was used in farming and changed at the genetic level through generations of selective breeding) by native farmers in prehistoric times, between seven thousand and twelve thousand years ago. More recently, extensive genetic modification has resulted in many varieties of corn. Over time, the plants' genes have been extensively modified, bringing us today's good-tasting, high-MSG corn.

In fact, twenty percent of the protein content of corn is glutamic acid—much of it is bound into protein and harmless, but some is not imprisoned in protein and is free to be absorbed quickly into the body.

Many of my patients were sensitive to corn, as I am. As with all increased-MSG foods, a limited amount of corn should not cause extreme symptoms in people sensitive to glutamic acid. Of course, people allergic to corn should avoid it. (It should be noted that corn, including corn on the cob, seems to be better tolerated if the kernels are boiled until soft and the boiling water then discarded.)

Quinoa

Quinoa belongs to the goosefoot family of plants, and although it contains gluten, it is not the type of gluten found in wheat, rye, barley, and oats. Thus, in theory, quinoa should be a good substitute for these grains for those people with sensitivities to gluten.

However, I believe that, similar to corn, it can cause symptoms in MSG-sensitive people. I have prepared quinoa for myself numerous times, varying every preparation step I could think of, including boiling time, and following every meal I suffered a sleepless night—a sure symptom to me of a high-MSG food. Because of my experience, I cannot advise quinoa for people sensitive to MSG.

Tomato/Potato

When tomatoes and potatoes were domesticated is unknown but over two thousand years ago they were already being cultivated in Mexico. Tomatoes and potatoes were originally derived from the same plant, with tomatoes growing among the leaves of the plant and potatoes growing underground in the roots.

Tomatoes and potatoes are known to contain a high level of the flavor enhancer, free glutamic acid, its sister amino acid aspartic acid, and also citric acid. The act of processing tomato products concentrates both the MSG and citrus content of tomatoes.

It is best not to indulge too heavily in tomatoes, especially processed tomatoes, and to use limited amounts of sliced tomato instead of processed tomato if you suffer from the aging chemicals.

Eating potatoes at frequent meals also allows the accumulation in your body of excess MSG, aspartic acid, and fruit acids such as citric acid.

Peanut

Archeologists have dated the oldest specimens of peanuts, found in Peru, to about 7,600 years ago. Since that time, the extended period of cultivation allowed farmers to continually plant the peanuts that tasted best. The peanuts that tasted best were those with high levels of free glutamic acid. Avoid or limit your intake of peanuts and peanut-containing products.

Foods That Naturally Contain High Levels of Free Glutamic Acid.
Fungus and Yeast Foods

Fungi, also referred to as yeasts and mold, are single-celled or many-celled organisms extensively used in food and drink preparations. Baker's yeast causes bread to rise, other yeasts ferment alcoholic beverages, and still others assist in making products such as soy sauce, sake, miso, and tempeh. Fungus and yeast have naturally high levels of free glutamic acid in their bodies and are often added to foods to improve the flavor of the foods.

Mushrooms

Some strains of fungus living in the ground extend these fleshy, spore-bearing fruiting bodies above ground to release into the air the spores that develop into new fungus. As they have a high content of free glutamic acid, avoid them and the foods they season.

Algae

Seaweed is the common name for a grass-like sea plant made up of multicellular marine algae. Seaweed was used for years to flavor foods and the reason for this improved taste was not known until MSG was isolated from the seaweed and identified as the flavor enhancer that causes such a remarkably improved taste in foods.

Extracts from seaweed, named "agar" and "carrageenan," are used in food manufacturing to keep mixed ingredients from separating and give foods a smooth texture. Commercial preparations of agar and carrageenan may contain free amino acids including both aspartic and glutamic acid. Even though both amino acids are regarded as harmless, if you have issues with MSG sensitivity you should avoid or limit foods that contain agar and carrageenan.

Joanne K. Tobacman, associate professor of clinical medicine at the University of Chicago, has studied carrageenan and is concerned. She notes that carrageenan has been used in laboratory animals to induce inflammation, the same chronic inflammation that is a cause of heart disease, Alzheimer's, Parkinson's, and cancer. Many food products contain carrageenan and, depending on the foods you include in your diet, your exposure may be higher than you think.

You will find seaweed or its derivatives, carrageenan and agar, on the list of ingredients of many foods made from milk, like yogurt, ice cream, and cottage cheese. They are found in jelly, chocolate, and salad dressing, as well as in pie filling and processed meats, where they are used as a fat substitute. Read the label of any of these foods carefully and decide whether you want to consume them.

Foods and Drinks That Contain High Levels of Free Glutamic Acid Because of Fermentation, Autolysis, and Proteolysis

I have pointed out how mold and yeast are used to ferment alcoholic beverages, such as beer, wine, and whiskey, and soy products, such as tofu and soy sauce, and how this fermentation increases the content of free glutamic acid. Bacteria can be added to the list of organisms

35

used in fermentation, especially in the creation of cheeses. The foods they ferment contain protein and the fermentation process splits apart the protein, freeing the bound amino acids, including glutamic acid, to enter the fermenting solution,

As mentioned, the microorganisms doing the fermenting also contain significant levels of free glutamic acid inside their cells. When these microorganisms die and disintegrate they release their content of potent digestive enzymes and these enzymes further degrade proteins to amino acids—a process called self-digestion or "autolysis." Therefore, autolysis increases the content of free amino acids, including free glutamic acid in the form of MSG, in the food. This increased content is signified on food labels as "autolyzed yeast extract."

The breaking down of protein into amino acids by an outside source (as opposed to degradation due to death) is called "proteolysis" and the chemicals that promote proteolysis are present in many organisms including yeast, bacteria, plants, and animals. Several commercial products are available that use proteolysis to tenderize tough meat fibers, including papain from the papaya, bromelain from pineapple and actinidin from the kiwi fruit. If you suffer from MSG sensitivity, it is best to completely avoid meat tenderized with these proteolytic chemicals, as the levels of MSG may be more than you can tolerate.

To make a long story short, every fermented product contains MSG. The higher the content of protein was in the food being fermented, the higher the content of MSG there will be in the fermented food or beverage. Because cereal grains such as wheat and barley are mainly carbohydrates and contain lesser amounts of protein, they release less MSG than protein-heavy milk or soybeans. High-protein content is why soy and milk proteins are so frequently used in the industrial production of MSG. Fermentation and autolysis also explain why cheese, especially the well-aged cheeses, contains so much MSG. When you think of cheese, think of MSG.

Products That Contain High Levels of Free Glutamic Acid Because of Hydrolysis

"Hydrolysis" is the breaking apart of protein by boiling it in special solutions, thus freeing glutamic acid from the protein and turning it into free MSG. The "freed" MSG is then collected and added to foods that do not contain large quantities of MSG. (A note: hydrolysis is often confused with "hydrogenation." Hydrogenation, however, happens to fats and oils, not proteins, and is not examined in this book.)

Check the list of ingredients on any food to see if a "hydrolyzed protein" (such as hydrolyzed soy or milk protein) has been added to the food product you are considering buying. If so, don't buy it.

Hydrolysis also breaks down the protein in meat into amino acids, resulting in gelatin that is rich in the glutamic acid that was once imprisoned in the animal protein. So you should probably also avoid products containing gelatin.

Food processors list MSG on the list of ingredients on the label if they use it in its pure form. However, they do not need to note it on the label if they add it in the form of a product that already contains large amounts of MSG such as hydrolyzed protein, autolyzed yeast, Parmesan cheese, or "natural flavoring." This kind of labelling is a common practice, which is why you must know these sources of MSG to avoid eating and drinking them.

Products That Are Simply Concentrated MSG

The final source of MSG in the diet is the glutamic acid manufactured by hydrolysis and autolysis, combined with an ion such as sodium, calcium, or magnesium, and then dried. When you see monosodium glutamate on the label, you know that the food manufacturer is being honest about what the food contains. You can applaud them for their honesty, but you still should not buy the product.

Part 6:
A List of Ingredients on Food Labels That Signify the Presence (or Possible Presence) of MSG

Having discussed how MSG enters our diet, let us look at the following lists. I developed these lists as I identified the foods that caused my patients' symptoms, and that also affected me. I also included information found on many websites, including www.truthinlabeling.org/hiddensources.html, which was established by Adie and Jack Samuels.

Although I have no relationship with them other than discussing MSG sensitivity with Adie while researching this present book, I do know that Jack passed away; he was severely sensitive to even a minute amount of MSG—a degree of sensitivity that I have encountered in other patients. These days, Adie maintains the website and told me that she developed her list using information from MSG-sensitive people and from studies about MSG found in some medical literature. I do not know if there is a better source of MSG information than these sources. In fact, my own research of the medical literature made me wish that there were more studies of the amount of free glutamic acid in the food we eat.

If a Food Label Contains These Ingredients, You Should Avoid It

If the label on any food or beverage lists one of the following, it means it definitely includes free glutamic acid:
- monosodium glutamate
- monopotassium glutamate
- calcium glutamate
- monoammonium glutamate
- magnesium or natrium glutamate

If a Food Label Contains These Ingredients, You Should

Probably Avoid It

The following foods and beverages are likely to include free glutamic acid, and so you are best served if you avoid them:

- Any fermented food or beverage, including:
  - bean-based manufactured products (soy sauce, tofu, soy milk, etc.)
  - manufactured dairy products (cheese, yogurt, etc.)
  - processed fruit-based products (wine, brandy, etc.)
  - processed grain-based products (alcoholic beverages such as beer, whiskey, etc.)
- Any food or beverage containing autolyzed ingredients, including:
  - yeast
  - yeast extract
  - yeast food
  - yeast nutrient
  - torula
  - brewer's yeast
- Any food or beverage containing hydrolyzed ingredients including any kind of plant or vegetable protein
- Any food or beverage containing protein which has been altered in any way, including:
  - protein fortified
  - calcium caseinate or sodium caseinate
  - gelatin
  - meat tenderized with papain, bromelain, or actinidin
  - soy protein, soy protein concentrate, or soy protein isolate
  - textured protein
  - whey protein, whey protein concentrate, or wheat protein isolate
- Any food containing enzymes or proteases

If a Food Label Contains These Ingredients, You Should

Avoid or Limit Them in Your Diet:

- Any "flavors" or "flavoring," including any natural flavor that does not identify the source of the flavoring (remember: MSG is a "natural" flavoring)
- Any food or beverage labeled "ultra-pasteurized"
- Any malted or sprouted seed, including barley malt or almond milk
- Bouillon and broth
- Pectin
- "Seasonings" that are not listed out
- Stock

Natural Foods That Should Be Avoided or Limited in Your Diet:

The following natural foods are also high in free glutamic acid, so you should minimize their use in your diet:

- Seaweed (known as kelp and other names) and its products carrageenan and agar
- Lightly cooked corn and corn products, including corn syrup
- Peanuts and peanut products
- Quinoa
- Tomatoes, especially concentrated tomato products

Part 7:
Summary

If you are sensitive to MSG, reducing the amount you consume can relieve chronic, irritating, and often painful symptoms. It can relieve your distressing constipation or subdue your painful migraines or cluster headaches—or, as in my case, allow you to enjoy restful sleep and awake refreshed. If it helps you recover your memory and your ability to take care of yourself, what a blessing it will be; after all, although discomfort, pain, and sleeplessness are distressing, mental deterioration is far worse. Much worse.

Of secondary—but still pleasing—importance: after years of hammering your taste buds with MSG, avoiding it awakens your taste buds to the great flavors in foods you thought had little or no taste. For example, even if you always enjoyed the crunching sensation of celery, now you will taste flavors in celery that you have never experienced. No matter what food you eat, whether meat, vegetable, or fruit, your awakened sense of taste will bring you delight. And, you may learn to flavor foods with the spices our ancestors used before we started to depend on MSG to flavor our foods.

The third factor that will make you feel good about reducing the MSG in your diet: you do not need to completely eliminate MSG, you need only to reduce how much you eat to the amount you can tolerate. Unfortunately, how much MSG you can tolerate cannot be predicted; you will have to develop a sense of how much MSG-flavored food you can allow in your diet. This amount will most likely be different from what your brother, your best friend, and your neighbor across the street can tolerate.

To understand this, remember that, as we age, many of our genes also age and the switches that control their power are progressively lowered. These genes and their switches maintain the enzymes that allow us to tolerate MSG. With age, the switches dim (like a dining room light on a slowly turning dimmer switch). Your ability to consume MSG depends on how much your MSG dimmer switch has been dimmed.

Even though you do not need to eliminate MSG from your diet completely, you still must be careful of how much you consume. Remember that the effects of excess MSG last for three days—it takes three days to eliminate the excess from your body. If you eat small excesses of MSG-containing foods for two to three consecutive days, the MSG in the meal on the third day may combine with the MSG from previous meals to precipitate headaches, diarrhea, or other symptoms. It is best to prevent these symptoms by following a low-MSG diet.

Always consume alcohol in moderation and with the understanding that every alcoholic beverage adds to the total MSG you are consuming.

As for me, I dread the onset of the mental deterioration that can accompany aging. I know that any foods that contain the aging chemicals injure and destroy nerves and hasten the onset of this horrible deterioration. Any day that you or I consume a diet low in these chemicals that age us is a day that we are resisting the aging of our brains.

It is never too late to reduce or eliminate MSG from your diet. You can recover much of the youth you have lost, the ability to think, and the gift of remembering. You now know my story, and that this is possible—I am the proof. Just do not wait too long to start.

Chapter 4

Low-Calorie Sweeteners—the MSG "Wannabes"

In this discussion of low-calorie sweeteners (LCS), I will use aspartic acid, one of the body's amino acids, as representative of the group of LCS, mainly because it is the sweetener that, from my practice, I know best. I place other low-calorie sweeteners in the LCS category with aspartic acid because so many of my patients—especially those with migraine and cluster headaches—lost their symptoms when they stopped using all LCS.

Once headaches stopped, we never further investigated the effect of each individual LCS on symptoms such as headaches or abdominal distress. I could not have undertaken these studies if I had wanted to; after all, my patients would not have agreed to trial doses of different types of LCS to see which caused their headaches—and I would never have asked them to do so.

So if I am being unkind to any low-calorie sweeteners that do not cause symptoms, I sincerely apologize. But, for our discussion, I will use aspartic acid to discuss the reactions to the low-calorie food chemicals in our diet that taste sweet.

How Aspartic Acid Is Related to MSG

Aspartic acid is one of the amino acids that make the proteins in our foods. When we eat these foods, our digestive systems break down these food proteins to amino acids that then recombine to make the proteins in the genes, nerves, muscles, and organs throughout our bodies. We have already spent much time discussing MSG because understanding this diet chemical helps us understand the other aging chemicals, including aspartic acid, so you already know much of how this works. Like glutamic acid, aspartic acid is not only an essential component of our proteins; it also— like MSG—is a neurotransmitter and neurotoxin.

Therefore, most of what I taught you about free glutamic acid (MSG) also applies to aspartic acid, with certain differences—mainly concerning the ability of these amino acids to harm sensitive sufferers. If we compared the harm caused by MSG with the harm caused by aspartic acid, MSG's power for harm would tower over aspartic acid like a beetle towers over an ant. If aspartic acid shared our drive and ambitions, it would detest being compared to MSG. It may desire a role as important as MSG, but it lacks some of MSG's potency and cunning.

An example of this potency is MSG's ability to powerfully stimulate and damage nerves. Aspartic acid probably has this same ability but, again, is less powerful. As an example of cunning, MSG hides under many different names in foods; aspartic acid hides in few foods and—if added as a chemical to a food or drink—its name must be acknowledged on the label. In other words, if you are paying attention, you know when you are consuming it. In fact, the name of the food we eat and the beverage we drink typically mentions the presence of a low-calorie sweetener if it contains it, a name such as "diet soda pop" or "low-calorie ice cream."

Further, while glutamic acid serves as a major neurotransmitter and neurotoxin, aspartic acid serves a more minor role.

Aspartic Acid in the Diet

To sweeten foods and drinks, food producers use aspartic acid in the form of aspartame, which is a combination of the amino acids aspartic acid and phenylalanine. They use aspartame to sweeten many foods and drinks, including chewing gum, dessert mixes, frozen desserts, pudding, soft drinks, and yogurt. They also provide it in dry form in tabletop sweeteners for consumers to use in foods. And even some cough drops and vitamins contain aspartame.

Who Says Aspartame Is Safe?

Many people who speak for aspartame regard it as safe. They point out that more than 200 studies have examined its safety. These studies have concluded that it does not cause headaches, seizures, Alzheimer's disease, Parkinson's disease, lupus, or multiple sclerosis. Further, no unsafe health consequences of aspartame have been conclusively identified.

The Reason I Disagree

My experiences have led me to fear that aspartame is not safe. I believe it is especially unsafe in patients sensitive to the aging chemicals. My experience with patients suffering headaches clearly points to aspartame as a cause. Many of these patients came to me knowing that low-calorie sweeteners such as those found in diet drinks set off vicious headaches. Other patients were unaware of this source of pain and found that removing diet drinks, low-calorie candy, and low-calorie processed foods gave many of them great relief. Seeing their lives get so much better served as an unmistakable sign to me that my patients suffered from the effects of the aging chemicals and told me that I must work to instruct them to be very careful of the other aging chemicals.

This experience in headache control prompted me to write about the food chemicals in my book Treating Sinus, Migraine and Cluster Headaches, My Way. Once I helped my patients understand the headache causes, which were lurking in their homes and in the atmosphere, told them about the food allergy causes, and counseled them on their diets, I was able to relieve many of the headaches my patients suffered.

Aspartic Acid in Natural Foods

As I wrote this book, I became more and more convinced that what we call "natural" foods, such as wheat and corn, have been extensively modified over thousands of years and are, in fact, genetically altered by their growers' efforts. Though I will continue to use the term "natural" to differentiate unprocessed foods from processed foods, in my mind the exact meaning of natural has become unclear.

Nature used both aspartic and glutamic acid in the proteins that make our foods. However, the amount of aspartic acid in our natural foods is markedly lower than the amount of glutamic acid. Glutamic acid usually makes up about 10% of the proteins in foods. In corn, milk, and soy its level reaches about 20%; in gluten, it reaches an even higher level—evidence that farmers in ancient and modern times extensively modified corn, soy, and gluten from the probable 10% glutamic acid level of the original ancestral plants.

The story is much different with aspartic acid. It reaches its peak level at a little over 10% of protein in alfalfa and corn, and in wheat its level is low—only about 6 percent. I wondered why farmers did not modify these foods to increase their aspartic acid content, and I found the answer in body builders' comments about using aspartic acid as a supplement to increase the efficiency of exercising. Those who commented on its taste described it as being unpleasant, even "awful." Farmers, being practical and intelligent, did not force more aspartic acid into their crops because there was no advantage to having more of this bad-tasting amino acid than the amount originally planned by nature.

If aspartic acid wanted to be the kingpin neurostimulant and neurotoxin, dethroning glutamic acid, it couldn't. It remained a wannabe.

Where Aspartic Acid May Be Important

I noted in our discussion of glutamic acid that it is not the bound glutamic acid in protein that causes symptoms but the glutamic acid that has been freed from protein. It is the same with glutamic acid's close relative, aspartic acid.

Besides being added to processed foods, where the addition of aspartic acid is noted on the label, this amino acid is also found in sprouting seeds often found in health food stores. Unfortunately, these sprouting seeds include such foods as otherwise healthy quinoa, rice, and corn.

In the process of sprouting, the seed releases both glutamic and aspartic acids from their prisons in protein, converting them into free amino acids able to nourish the growing plant. These same free amino acids may affect people sensitive to the aging food chemicals. I urge you to watch your intake of these seed foods, confining them to the amount you can tolerate without symptoms.

A Patient's Symptoms

I asked a patient to write the following letter (altered to respect her privacy) describing her experiences with low-calorie sweeteners. She later discovered that she also reacted to corn (by developing hives on her cheeks) and to MSG (with diarrhea).

> June 17, 1985
>
> Dear Doctor Walsh:
>
> With this [letter] I want to describe the problems I have had when I've had [a low-calorie dessert flavored with aspartame]. The first time, I suffered a reaction—when it first came out—which gave me a terrible headache soon after eating it. This headache did not get any better with aspirin or Tylenol.

> [In] the second episode, last month, [I] reacted after only five sips of diet soda. I got shortness of breath, cold sweat, fast heart, and very panicky. These effects wore off after about two hours.
>
> Talking with my neighbor, who is now pregnant— [I found out that] her OB doctor recommended not drinking anything with [a low-calorie sweetener flavored with aspartame].

Without a doubt, my patient suffers from a sensitivity to low-calorie sweeteners. Both MSG and aspartame, two of the aging food chemicals, cause her headaches. I showed you the letter not to describe an unusual history of a patient with headaches, but to describe a usual history. This patient diagnosed the cause of her headaches before coming to me for evaluation; as I already mentioned, many, many of my patients also recognized that low-calorie sweeteners caused their headaches before seeing me.

In patients whose self-diagnosis was so accurate, I could not add to their knowledge of the low-calorie sweeteners. I was able to contribute to their care by expanding their knowledge of the other aging food chemicals—chemicals that would be expected to cause similar symptoms. Further, when talking to this patient I made sure that she knew that a food allergy can cause similar headaches to those caused by the aging food chemicals and she has, since, tested positive to a corn allergy, so she will watch to see if corn causes her any additional distress. Utilizing the above clues in planning her diet helped prevent future headaches.

Although her letter is short, it contains other excellent information. Notice her symptoms: "shortness of breath, cold sweat, fast heart, and very panicky." These are symptoms shared by many of my patients. I have mentioned repeatedly that the aging chemicals attack nerves; her symptoms indicate her head pain arises from affected nerves in the head. They also indicate activation of the "fight-or-flight" or "acute stress" response mediated by the autonomic nervous system, which can result in shortness of breath, cold sweat, a fast heartbeat, and panic. All these symptoms show the power of the aging food chemicals—in this case caused by low-calorie sweeteners—to irritate a person's nerves.

Another nugget of information held in this short letter is the speed of the diet soda reaction. I have been stressing that food sensitivity is a slowly plodding beast that only starts after a quantity of food chemical is ingested that is more than the sensitive person can tolerate. Five sips of diet pop is hardly a large amount and the resultant rapid attack is in no way slow. This is an illustration of how—if a person is sensitive enough, in a reactive state, and eats or drinks a sensitizing chemical—the reaction can be as quick as the strike of a poisonous snake.

Finally, I agree with her neighbor's pregnancy doctor: low-calorie sweeteners truly are poor choices during pregnancy.

Chapter 5

Gluten—the Infamous Food Chemical

Gluten sensitivity, though I have been working with it for many years, is finally in the news. After years of treating patients who were unaware that they were gluten sensitive, after years of wandering the grocery aisles looking for gluten-free foods and finding few, and after years of asking for a gluten-free menu at restaurants and encountering blank stares from servers, gluten is finally receiving the attention it deserves. Finally, many people are aware they suffer gluten sensitivity. I find shelves of gluten-free foods in stores. Servers immediately bring me the gluten-free menu when asked. What a wonderful change—gluten is now infamous.

What Is Gluten?

You may be aware that gluten is a major protein in the grains of the grass family (wheat, rye, barley, and oats). This protein is "sticky" and wheat gluten is used in the baking industry to hold together bread, pastries, and other grain products. Because gluten has been in the news so often, you may be aware that many people believe they suffer health complications caused by gluten. You or a loved one may also be suffering from symptoms that you suspect are caused by gluten and, if you do suspect it, there is a good chance you are right. In this chapter I will endeavor to increase your knowledge of gluten, its potential for causing harm to susceptible people, and how you can avoid it if it harms you.

Many experts question whether oat gluten causes symptoms for gluten-sensitive people. (I believe it does and they should avoid or reduce their consumption of products made from oats.) Corn also contains gluten, but not the same gluten as in the grass grains. Although many experts on celiac disease regard corn gluten as acceptable for their patients, I suspect—but cannot prove—that many patients sensitive to gluten in the grains of the grass family also react to corn gluten, just not as severely as they react to the gluten of wheat, rye, barley, and oats.

My Personal Discovery of Gluten

I do not criticize other doctors for not realizing how many patients suffer gluten sensitivity. Even though I specialized in evaluating and treating patients suffering from both food allergies and food sensitivities—and have authored and published books on food allergies and sensitivities—I must admit that I was slow to recognize how many of my patients suffer from sensitivity to gluten.

In researching my first book, published in 1991, Treating Food Allergy, My Way, I identified four of the six aging chemicals: MSG, sugar, citric acid, and low-calorie sweeteners. But I had not yet recognized that lactose and gluten belonged with these four. Nor did I make a clear distinction between a food allergy and a food sensitivity.

In my book published in 1993, Treating Sinus, Migraine and Cluster Headaches, My Way: An Allergist's Approach to Headache Treatment, I described the importance of food allergies in causing headaches. However, I did not recognize the critical importance of food sensitivities. Instead I attributed to "delayed food allergy" the headaches caused by food sensitivity.

It was only in my most recent book, published in 2000, Food Allergies: The Complete Guide to Understanding and Relieving Your Food Allergies that I focused more heavily on the chemicals in foods, again discussing MSG, sugar, citric acid, and low-calorie sweeteners. Again I underestimated the contribution of lactose and gluten and did not clearly indicate that the chemicals of the gluten syndrome caused food sensitivity and not food allergy.

Food Allergy Versus Food Sensitivity

With this book I am attempting to clear up the confusion between food sensitivities and food allergies, and to present to you a more complete picture of the sensitivity to the aging chemicals so common in our diet. I want to help you find and eat foods that are less threatening. I have already discussed the differences between a food allergy and a food sensitivity, especially the sensitivity to the aging chemicals. Now is a good time to briefly restate these differences:

The Basic Cause

An overactive immune system causes food allergies; aging and weakening of the action of the genes controlling the digestion and processing of food causes sensitivity to the aging chemicals.

The Mediators of Harm

The immune system releases antibodies that cause symptoms in reaction to a food allergy. Consuming the excess aging chemicals found in our modern diet damages and destroys our nerves and damages our brain.

The Result of Harm

In a food allergy, the antibodies cause symptoms such as sneezing, wheezing, and itching. In sensitivity to the aging chemicals, the food chemicals injure nerves, the act of which results in the malfunction of body systems, yielding symptoms of aging such as confusion and memory loss, and pain such as the throbbing of headaches.

Amounts Needed to Activate Symptoms

In a food allergy, a small amount of food can bring rapid-acting symptoms. In a food sensitivity, much larger amounts are necessary because the ability to digest and process the troublesome diet chemicals is not gone, it is only diminished. Because of this, the symptoms typically appear only after excess consumption of these chemicals.

Difficulty in Diagnosis

A food allergy can be readily diagnosed by skin and blood tests. Sensitivity to the aging chemicals cannot be diagnosed by tests; it is only diagnosed by the symptoms the sufferers experience and by the relief of symptoms provided by elimination diets.

The Cause of Gluten Sensitivity

Briefly stated, gluten is a food that introduces excess MSG into the diet. This means that gluten sensitivity is also MSG sensitivity.

Now you know why MSG had to be discussed before putting gluten under our magnifying glass. I could have included gluten in the chapter on MSG. However, because wheat, rye, barley, and oats form such an important part of our diet, gluten sensitivity deserves a chapter of its own.

Indications That MSG Is the Cause of Gluten Sensitivity

The strongest indications that MSG is the cause of gluten's symptoms are the symptoms of my own patients. Once I became aware of the surprising number of gluten-sensitive patients, I quickly learned that I could not diagnose my patients as gluten sensitive if they were not also sensitive to MSG. Without MSG sensitivity, I felt uncomfortable diagnosing gluten sensitivity. In almost all cases, my patients' sensitivity to MSG usually became apparent some years before the gluten sensitivity.

The second indication that MSG is the cause of gluten sensitivity is the surprising amount of glutamic acid in gluten. This dangerous amino acid, glutamic acid, is present and abundant in most proteins, usually forming about 10% of the protein. In some proteins, including milk, corn, and soy, its levels are as high as about 20%. In wheat gluten, however, its level soars to even higher levels of the protein.

When you consider the large amount of glutamic acid in gluten it is easy to realize how it causes symptoms, especially if the glutamic acid—which is loosely held in the gluten protein—escapes from the gluten protein quickly when eaten, and is absorbed into the body quickly. This rapid absorption, in sensitive people, overwhelms the weakened systems that release this powerful amino acid from the nerve synapse.

The third indication that MSG sensitivity and gluten sensitivity are the same is that they share the same symptoms. These symptoms are wide-ranging and include those below:

» Abdominal distention	» Hives
» Abdominal pain and cramping	» Joint pain
» Bloating	» Nausea
» Borborygmi (stomach rumbling)	» Sweating, chills, clamminess, and dizziness (the same symptoms as hypoglycemia)
» Constipation	
» Diarrhea	» Vomiting
» Fatigue	» Weight loss (unexplained)
» Headaches, migraines	

Why the Symptoms Are So Diverse

You will be tempted to think: "This is not right. There are too many symptoms here; no medical condition can cause all of these symptoms. Aren't these people who claim they suffer from gluten sensitivity imagining them?" The answer is no, these symptoms are all real, are caused by the aging chemicals, and are not a figment of the sufferers' imaginations.

What unites all these symptoms is that they have a single cause: injured nerves. The increased concentration of the neurotransmitter, free glutamic acid, around stimulated nerves causes this injury. This corrosive chemical damages the nerves controlling many of our body's systems such as the brain, intestine, and skin, leading to this multiplicity of symptoms.

In my practice, while treating allergies, it became obvious to me that my patients did not suffer symptoms that were identical. I wondered why they experienced different symptoms, thinking that they should share the same symptoms. For instance, Mary had migraine headaches, Jack was constipated, Kay and Jim felt very bloated, and Betty suffered all of these symptoms. Why did Jack, Kay and Jim not also suffer migraine headaches? I believe the answer lies in our genes.

The Human Genome Project found about twenty to thirty thousand genes and Mary, Jack, Kay, Jim, and Betty have many gene differences that must make them especially susceptible to different symptoms. The Human Genome Project also found that "switches" control the power of genes. These switches slow, weaken, or dim the genes' actions and there are many switches dispersed among the genes. As we age, many of these switches seriously hamper or weaken the removal of MSG from around the nerves. Which switches are affected can differ between people and most likely are different in Mary, Jack, Kay, Jim, and Betty and account for some of the differences in their symptoms.

So the diversity of symptoms in gluten-sensitive people is not surprising. This diversity of symptoms is to be expected.

What Is Celiac Disease and Why Must We Examine It Now?

Let me answer the second question first. Celiac disease and sensitivity to the aging chemicals are similar because they both involve gluten. However, there are differences and these differences are important. They permit those who suffer from food chemical sensitivity to eat foods prohibited to the celiac patient. The celiac diet is very strict; our diet is more relaxed. The diets must be different because the conditions are different, as is shown below.

The Surface Lining of the Intestine

Celiac disease: When they eat gluten, Celiac sufferers' own immune systems attack the lining of their small intestine. The attack centers on the area of the intestine packed with tufts of hair-like strands called "villi." Normally, food going through the intestine gets trapped in these tufts, which process and absorb it. When the immune system attacks, that attack levels these tufts, replacing them with a smooth surface, which, like tile, does not allow food to cling to it and inhibits absorption of the food.

Sensitivity to the aging chemicals, on the other hand, does not attack the intestinal lining, so absorption of food is not diminished.

Diagnosis by Lab Tests and Intestinal Biopsy

Celiac disease: Doctors diagnose it by laboratory tests of the immune system and intestinal biopsy.

Sensitivity to the aging chemicals: Doctors cannot diagnose it by lab tests, intestinal biopsy, or x-ray.

Symptoms of Celiac Disease and Gluten Sensitivity

Celiac disease: As a result of the destruction of the villi, infants can suffer chronic diarrhea, swollen belly, pain, and failure to thrive. Older children are often overweight; some may suffer diarrhea, constipation, delayed puberty, and/or neurological symptoms. Adults usually display no digestive symptoms although many have weight loss. Other symptoms include anemia, skin rash with blistering and itch, headaches, joint pain, heartburn, and dental damage.

Sensitivity to the aging chemicals: As already mentioned, symptoms occur in many body systems due to damage to the nerves controlling those body systems.

Consequences of Celiac Disease and Sensitivity to the Aging Chemicals

Celiac disease: Scientists have been able to identify very threatening consequences of untreated celiac disease. These include malnutrition, bone loss, infertility, and neurological symptoms including numbness, tingling in the extremities, and balance loss. Untreated celiac disease patients may also face an increased threat of certain cancers.

Sensitivity to the aging chemicals: Symptoms are detailed in the chart above. In general, symptoms are more pain and discomfort than the more serious symptoms that accompany celiac disease in adults. However, the prolonged damage to and destruction of nerves in this disorder due to the aging chemicals may have tragic consequences including deterioration of the brain and body caused by prolonged nerve damage and destruction.

Lactose Sensitivity

(This will be discussed in depth, later in the text)

Celiac disease: Lactose sensitivity occurs as a result of impaired digestion because of villi destruction.

Sensitivity to the aging chemicals: Lactose sensitivity results from aging and dimming of genes.

Treatment of Celiac Disease and Gluten Sensitivity

Celiac disease: The highlight of treatment is complete, compulsive gluten avoidance.

Sensitivity to the aging chemicals: In the absence of studies showing severe damage from the diet—except for nerve damage leading to Alzheimer's disease and other neurological diseases—treatment consists of lowering the patient's consumption of the diet chemicals to an amount that can be tolerated.

Let me reemphasize: I believe that sensitivity to the aging chemicals is best understood as caused by the aging and weakening of the actions of genes. It cannot be diagnosed by laboratory tests or biopsy and, therefore, no long-term peer-reviewed studies are currently able to tell us the long-term consequences of this syndrome except for the already known effects they have on a patient's nerves. Hopefully, no further threatening consequences exist; the nerve involvement is enough to worry about. (If any evidence of immune system attack in sensitivity to the aging chemicals is found, my relaxed approach to treatment will have to be revisited.)

Now that we have examined gluten, low-calorie sweeteners, and MSG, it is time to tell you about another troublesome food chemical, a very important chemical: refined sugar.

Chapter 6
Refined Sugar—the "H" Food Chemical (Heavy and Hyper)

What Is Refined Sugar?

Refined sugar is the sugar you spoon into your coffee, mix with flour to make sweet treats, and find on the label of many processed meats. It comes mainly from three sources: beet sugar from sugar beets, cane sugar from sugar cane, and corn sugar from corn. Beet and cane sugars are called "sucrose" and corn sugar is often called "high-fructose corn syrup." Since the chemical compositions of the sucrose in cane sugar and beet sugar, and high-fructose corn sugar are practically identical, we will treat them all as identical for our discussion.

Brown sugar is refined sugar mixed with molasses. Molasses is also a sugar, as are fruit nectars, cane juice, honey, and agave nectar—all of which are added to processed foods to sweeten them. As a group, on labels they are referred to as "added sugars."

Sucrose and high-fructose corn sugar are composed of two simple sugars, glucose and fructose, bonded together. They taste sweet because of the high concentration of their fructose content, which is much sweeter than glucose.

On the other hand, in many foods naturally rich in sugar, such as potatoes or bread, the sugar is composed mainly of glucose and does not have the sweet taste of foods containing higher levels of fructose.

Many fruits naturally contain elevated levels of fructose, including: grapes, bananas, mangos, sweet cherries, apples, pineapples, pears, and kiwi fruit. Because their fructose content is so high, people striving to reduce their intake of fructose should not eat these fruits in excess.

I believe one apple and one pear a day should be tolerable with a small amount of other fruits. At least these fruits also deliver other healthy nutrients. However, juices made from these fruits concentrate the sugars of these fruits and can add even more fructose to the diet. With fruit juice, you can quickly exceed your tolerance for fructose, so it is probably best to avoid packaged fruit juices.

Now let's turn our attention to why we worry so much about refined sugar—which I call the "heavy" and "hyper" food chemical.

The First "H"—Heavy

By using the term "heavy," I acknowledge refined sugar's great power to make us heavy—or obese. But heavy also can be used to signify another power of refined sugar, the power of fructose to play, as in a movie, the "heavy" or villain. I consider refined sugar in our diet to play the role of the villain.

I am worried about refined sugar's villainous tendencies for what I consider to be a number of good reasons, the best of which is that the sugar harms us in a sneaky way because of a mistake in logic made by many people—including my fellow medical doctors. In their well-meaning fight against obesity, diabetes, and heart disease, many doctors incriminated the wrong foods. In the past they blamed fatty foods such as eggs and the fat in meats such as beef and pork for causing obesity and heart disease, while failing to implicate one of the real culprits: refined sugars. Now, many of today's medical researchers are reexamining these thoughts. They industriously seek out sugar's role in causing many common conditions including the above-mentioned obesity, plus diabetes and heart disease.

My Experience with Refined Sugar

To help you understand my feelings about sugar, let me tell you about my own experience with it. I am a typical sufferer from the aging chemicals. Therefore, I can use what I learned from my experiences with these chemicals to help you understand the harm they cause. If you are susceptible to the impact of the aging chemicals on your body and brain—and you continue to follow our modern diet—I believe you will suffer the same harm I experienced (and still do experience). If you are similarly sensitive, I want to lead you away from certain foods and guide you toward eating a diet that will preserve your youth, reverse some of the harm caused to your nerves, and improve your health.

I reacted to sugar: I was obese. At one time I was five feet eight inches tall and weighed two hundred and fifty pounds. Heavy? My suits had to be extra large.

I knew I had to lose weight but I knew I lacked the willpower to follow a strict weight-loss diet; I had to find another road to rid myself of fat. I decided that the road I could follow was to change one aspect of my diet—I could eliminate refined sugar. So, I did. I ate as much unsweetened food as I wanted, as often as I wanted. I lost about five pounds a year, year after year, until my weight dropped to two hundred pounds. I was pleased.

Then, some years later, I began to identify the other aging food chemicals that were causing my patients to suffer chronic illness and I changed my diet to avoid these foods, as well. Slowly my weight lessened even further as I lost a further forty pounds. I did all of this while never limiting my intake of food, never denying myself as much as I wanted to eat, and seldom being hungry. All together, just through this diet modification, I have lost eighty pounds!

This diet ended my bloated feeling as my weight dropped, correlating with what I observed in my patients: they could lose weight as long as they changed their diet to reduce their intake of the aging chemicals, especially refined sugar.

Then, two patients suffering headaches startled me with their comments. Both were following my diet guidelines, and both returned to my office in the same week. Both mentioned that the diet quieted their headaches. They also told me how much better they felt as their bloating and abdominal distress subsided. Then, they both said, in about the same words, "And I lost thirty pounds!"

From their expressions, I could tell that this weight loss startled them as much as their comments startled me. Their experience of lessening bloating and losing weight coincided exactly with mine. This coincidence of two women losing the same amount of weight, telling me about it in the same words—and in the same week— brought the relationship between bloating and obesity forcibly to my attention.

Exploring the Current Studies on Refined Sugar

Current diet research is compatible with my experiences: you can expect weight loss if you avoid the food chemicals that cause aging, especially refined sugar. I have been following various medical studies for years, examining reports and listening to lectures by scientists. I strongly suggest you also become aware of this research by looking into the following references.

A summary of this research is provided by Gary Taubes and can be found in his book Why We Get Fat: And What to Do About It.

Taubes has spent years of journalistic research on diet and chronic diseases and I believe he writes with great authority. In his article for the New York Times magazine titled: "Is Sugar Toxic?" (New York Times, April 13, 2011), he discusses the evidence for this toxicity as he reviews a lecture given by Dr. Robert Lustig on May 26, 2009, titled "Sugar: The Bitter Truth."

Dr. Lustig is a pediatric obesity specialist and treats many obese children at his clinic at the University of California, San Francisco. His lectures have been very popular and millions visit his websites. Because he not only studies these issues, but also treats patients, he not only has theoretical knowledge of obesity through his research and teaching, but also has a practical understanding of obesity. In short, he is an expert.

In his discussion of refined sugar, Dr. Lustig calls it a "poison" and a "toxin" (the latter term I also use to describe the effects of the aging chemicals). I also believe that sugar is toxic to those patients who are sensitive to the aging chemicals, who eat and drink them in excess, and who suffer symptoms as described in this chapter. He does not limit his use of the term only to sugar's impact on sensitive people but believes that anyone who uses refined sugar in excess suffers toxicity. (He might be right.) He describes studies that show that this use is excessive in our modern diet, pointing out (each of which we will discuss more, below):

- Nobody chooses to be obese, to be diabetic, or to have heart disease.
- The consequences of consuming excess refined sugar are many, including obesity, diabetes, and heart disease.
- Glucose does not cause these consequences.
- Fructose, with excess intake, does cause obesity, diabetes, and heart disease.
- Excess refined sugar seriously reduces the power of the hormones that tell us that we have eaten enough food and are full.
- Eating less food does not eliminate refined sugar's threat if we continue to consume it.
- Eating the right foods does reduce the threat.
- Exercise improves muscle tone, health, and mental ability but does not counteract obesity.

Nobody Chooses to Be Obese, Diabetic, or Suffer Heart Disease

Let's tackle this thought first because I believe most people agree with it. The vast majority of obese people regret their obesity. Carrying excess weight is tiring, uncomfortable, and unhealthy. It subjects overweight children to bullying, subjects overweight adolescents to difficulty dating, and subjects overweight adults to distressing choices in clothing, all resulting from society's reaction to obesity. Nobody chooses to be overweight. But, unfortunately, they are stuck with obesity until they understand why they are obese and learn to live and eat in such a way that there is a chance for the pounds to drop away.

I believe this is true of the majority of people suffering from obesity but also realize that there are people who, because of mental or physical illness or genetic makeup, cannot lose their extra pounds. They should not be condemned by us but should be evaluated and treated by specialists in obesity.

As for people suffering heart disease or diabetes, none of them chose these illnesses. Knowing the dietary causes of these illnesses will help them fight them effectively.

The Modern Diet Contains Excess Refined Sugar

The following facts support this contention:

Gary Taubes points out in his New York Times magazine article that the U.S. Department of Agriculture estimated that in 1980 Americans were eating and drinking 75 pounds of refined sugar per person each year. By early 2000 we had increased our yearly intake of refined sugar to 90 pounds. With this rise, more of us became obese and diabetic.

In 1980, one in seven Americans suffered from obesity, while in early 2000 one in three Americans suffered from obesity. The United States went from 6 million diabetics in 1980 to 14 million diabetics in 2000. Although there are other factors that encourage the emergence of obesity and diabetes, this parallel rise in sugar intake, obesity, and diabetes strongly suggests they are related.

We Tolerate Glucose, and Use It for Energy Storage and Use

It is not the sugar called glucose that causes obesity, diabetes, and heart disease. Glucose is commonly found in fruits and vegetables, and also occurs naturally in large quantities in our bodies.

In refined sugars such as sucrose and high-fructose corn syrup, glucose enters our diet combined with fructose. Glucose provides the major source of our body's energy, which is used by every cell of our body. When we eat glucose-containing foods, the majority of the sugar travels to the cells throughout our bodies for their use. About 20 percent is stored in the liver in the form of glycogen that is readily converted into glucose to produce energy—a process which does not harm the body.

Fructose, in Excess, Promotes Obesity, Diabetes, and Heart Disease

When we eat or drink foods and beverages sweetened with refined sugar in the form of sucrose and high-fructose corn syrup, fructose and glucose are quickly absorbed into the body. The glucose is well tolerated, while the fructose is poorly tolerated.

In contrast to glucose, where every cell in the body can absorb and use it, fructose is mainly shunted into the liver because only the liver can metabolize it. When we have studied the effect of fructose in animals, it has been found that the liver turns much of the fructose into fat and, at the same time, increases the production of insulin until the animal reaches a stage where it cannot maintain the increased insulin production and becomes insulin resistant—or diabetic. This process—

so far studied mainly in animals—may help explain diabetes in humans.

With insulin resistance, triglycerides—which are thought to be a factor in narrowing cardiac blood vessels—increase, showing a possible pathway by which humans suffer heart disease from refined sugar.

The question arises: If fructose is so dangerous, why are we using it? The answers are multiple:

1) We thought fat, not sugar, was causing heart disease.

2) High-fructose corn syrup is cheap and plentiful.

3) Fructose is sweet—almost twice as sweet as glucose.

4) Few medical caregivers recognized the danger until recently.

Excess Refined Sugar Seriously Reduces the Hormone Signal That We Have Eaten Enough Food

In addition to causing diabetes, insulin resistance induced by excess fructose ingestion seriously increases the sensation of hunger and retards the sensation of feeling full. Three hormones control how we react to foods: ghrelin (which signals the brain that the body is hungry), leptin (which signals that enough food has been eaten), and insulin (a rise in which reinforces the signal that the body has eaten enough).

When we become resistant to insulin, this signal that we are full becomes less effective, causing insulin-resistant people to feel great hunger in spite of eating sufficient food. It causes them to overeat their foods, and to become obese. Combine constant hunger and overindulgence in sweet foods and beverages, with the fatty liver resulting from consuming fructose, and you can see how obesity can become worse and worse.

Eating Less Food Does Not Eliminate Refined Sugar's Threat

Although obese people can lose weight by starving themselves, they are not attacking the root causes of their obesity. Those causes include the aging chemicals. As long as the obese eat and drink them beyond the amount their bodies can tolerate, they will remain hungry and will not reach the state where they feel they have consumed enough food. Their feelings of fullness signaled by insulin and leptin will be weak. With this imbalance, and continual hunger, it is no wonder that, even if a diet is successful and someone loses weight, the lost weight returns easily. People in this situation will continue to suffer from obesity, diabetes, and heart disease.

Eating the Right Foods Does Reduce Refined Sugar's Threat

If you avoid or eliminate the foods and drinks with excess fructose, you can fight against the obesity, diabetes, and heart disease threat associated with refined sugar.

And, avoiding these chemicals is worthwhile. Removing the foods that degrade the satiety signaling (the signal which says that you are full) means that following a meal your stomach will feel pleasantly full; you will be far less tempted to overeat; and you will be more likely to lose weight. In fact, unless you have some complicating medical illness or a genetic constitution that prevents weight loss, or you stuff food into your mouth even though your body is signaling that you have eaten enough, you should be losing weight.

Although Exercise Improves Muscle Tone, Health, and Mental Ability, Exercise Does Not Counteract Obesity

This may be a difficult concept for you to accept, but let's try. If you use refined sugar to excess it will be hard for you to perform enough exercise to rid yourself of any weight gained as your liver turns the fructose into fat. You will carry this added fat while you exercise, making the exercise more exhausting.

To lose this fat while you continue to eat our modern diet you will need to exercise like a committed athlete, performing hours of moderate-to high-intensity exercise. If your exercise is less intense and prolonged, you will be left with the fat derived from the fructose you consumed. It takes hours of intense exercise to shed an appreciable amount of fat.

However, if you are a committed athlete, you should already know that you need glucose-based glycogen, not fructose-based fat, for energy storage and use during exercise. Both glucose and glycogen rapidly release energy during periods of intense exercise. Glucose acts like the gasoline that activates your car's motor; it rapidly changes to energy. That's why many pro athletes load up on glucose—not refined sugar—when they are doing carbohydrate loading.

Further, if you continue to eat processed sugar, your "I'm full" signals may not recover with exercise and you will still suffer hunger in spite of eating meals that should satisfy your hunger. If you succumb to the temptation to eat food and drink beverages with excess refined sugar, you will add more fat to your overburdened body.

These factors help explain why exercise, by itself, does not counteract obesity. However, exercise and changing your diet—especially eliminating the fructose of refined sugar—does counteract obesity. By avoiding fructose you can eat more energy-yielding glucose, add it to your energy stores as glycogen, and reactivate the satiety hormones. You should also feel comfortably full after each meal, be more active, and lose weight.

My Experience with Avoiding Excess Refined Sugar

My experience agrees with the concept that avoiding fructose-containing sweets also avoids accumulating fat with its accompanying weight gain. I can eat three meals a day and many snacks between meals and still lose weight. If I am hungry, I eat a between-meal snack. Following a full meal I feel content and do not want any food for hours. As long as I avoid refined sweets I do not miss these; on the other hand, if I eat even one bite I want more.

Additionally, in the past my blood pressure was elevated. After cutting out refined sugar, my blood pressure is now normal and I no longer take antihypertensive medicine.

All of these experiences are predicted by current research on carbohydrates, and if you follow my advice, you should experience the same results.

Where to Find Refined Sugar

Look for sugar on the list of ingredients printed on the labels of foods, and realize that many "natural" sugars are actually the results of genetic manipulation and processing. The ways that sugar can be noted are many, and might include (though this may not be a complete list):

- Any ingredient with the word "sugar" included (cane sugar, corn sugar, beet sugar)
- Any ingredient with the word "juice" included (fruit juice concentrate, fruit juice, cane juice)
- Any ingredient with the word "syrup" included (brown rice syrup, malt syrup, corn syrup, maple syrup)
- Agave
- Barley malt
- Caramel
- Dextrose
- Diastatic malt
- Fructose
- Galactose
- Glucose or glucose solids
- Golden syrup
- Honey
- Jaggery

- ☙ Lactose
- ☙ Maltodextrin
- ☙ Maltose
- ☙ Molasses
- ☙ Panela
- ☙ Panoche
- ☙ Rapadura
- ☙ Sucanat
- ☙ Sucrose
- ☙ Treacle

☙ As I mentioned, significant amounts of fructose are also found in our modern day fruits. Fruits, including apple, pear, and berries have been extensively modified from the original, natural fruits by being genetically selected for enlarged size and increased sweetness. With this genetic manipulation, the levels of fructose have been increased significantly in these formerly "natural" foods.

The Second "H"—Hyperactivity

We have spent much time examining the role of sugar in obesity and diabetes, the "heavy" of the title of this chapter. Now let's examine briefly how sugar causes hyperactivity.

Unfortunately, researchers can not agree on whether sugar causes hyperactivity. The doubters have studies that seem to support their contention that refined sugar does not cause hyperactivity. Some of these studies drew their conclusions by contrasting the behavior of two groups of children. One group was given sucrose (table sugar) and another group was given a low-calorie sweetener such as Aspartame (with the amino acid aspartic acid, a neurotoxin). The researchers noticed no difference in the activities of the two groups.

These studies either prove that sugar does not cause hyperactivity or that children suffer similar hyperactivity from both refined sugar and low-calorie sweeteners. Personally, I think the latter interpretation is correct. The fact that children react similarly to sugar and to a neurostimulant/neurotoxin such as aspartic acid strongly suggests that refined sugar has neurostimulant/neurotoxin actions, just like aspartic acid.

Further, looking at this similarity, I have come to strongly believe that refined sugar, itself, is a neurotoxin. Nerve stimulation and irritation are good explanations for the hyperactivity of children following sweet treats. A very wise elementary school teacher I know, Kevin, once remarked (and I paraphrase): "Thank goodness that this year there was no school the day after Halloween. With all that candy, the kids are uncontrollable!"

When I care for my grandchildren overnight I have learned to make a bargain with them. They can have a sugary treat but if they do they must go to bed on time. Without that bargain, I find it hard to slow them down enough to get them to bed.

These two examples, to me, are further proof that sugar causes hyperactivity. When we acknowledge the fact of hyperactivity being caused by a central nervous system toxic effect, the possibility that refined sugar is a neurotoxin is considerably enhanced.

I believe all of this is enough information to understand why you should consider avoiding refined sugar—and enough information to include refined sugar in the aging chemicals.

Chapter 7

Citric Acid—the Itchy Food Chemical (the First of the Aging Food Chemicals I Discovered)

I was serving in the United States Air Force after completing my medical internship and before my allergy residency. At that time, I was unsure of what field of medicine I would enter, even though I knew one of my choices was allergy treatment, and realized that this specialty attracted me because of my own allergies. With these thoughts in mind I was particularly interested in treating a little girl, Joyce (not her real name—and none of the names used in the following story are the people's real names), for a severe case of eczema. Unfortunately, my treatment was giving her little relief. Her skin was as red and raw as if it had been scraped with sandpaper. Her pain and itch were pitiful.

One day her father, Tony, brought her to my office and her skin was as soft and unmarked as a baby's skin. I said, "Well, finally my treatment is working. I am so glad!"

He replied, "Doctor Walsh, my wife and I appreciate your efforts to help our little girl but your directions really gave her little relief."

With my pride pretty deeply wounded, I asked. "Well, why is her skin so clear?"

He replied, "Because she treats herself! When her skin is severely broken out she draws her bath water, pours kitchen cleanser into it, and sits in it as she washes herself. Her bath ends her itch and her skin clears."

I had to believe her father; after all of medicine's conventional eczema treatments failed, he saw the kitchen cleanser curing her severe eczema. I was later to find that, indeed, our conventional treatments for eczema gave little help to my other eczema patients. Although my experience with Joyce taught me something new about eczema—something absent from the medical literature—I did not know what it was teaching me. Was I supposed to tell my eczema patients to wash themselves in kitchen cleanser? I really couldn't, because that would not be conventional treatment and, therefore, it was too much like medical experimentation and I would not subject them to experiments. What if the kitchen cleanser caused some harm?

But I knew that Joyce's story was trying to tell me something stunning about eczema so, even though I didn't know what it was trying to say, I never forgot Joyce's story. Her lesson was like a jigsaw puzzle with a vital piece missing, a piece that would tell me more about eczema than all my medical books—a piece that I was sure could tell me how to treat the miserably itchy skin rash.

I found that missing puzzle piece years later, after my fellowship in allergy at the Mayo Clinic, while practicing as an allergy specialist. Another child supplied it, a boy, and this time his mother, not his father, supplied the information. It was—to me—information so radical, so stunning, and so useful that it unlocked the secret to the treatment of many cases of eczema.

I liked his mother; she was an intelligent and honest person and a great mother to her son, Craig. Like my previous patient, Joyce, he was a child with severe eczema. His skin, also like Joyce's, was red and raw and obviously extremely irritated.

I still can picture Craig's mother in my mind and remember our conversation and it went like this: "Mary, our treatment really does not help Craig, does it?"

"No, it doesn't."

Still looking for that piece of the jigsaw puzzle, I asked her, "Do you have any feeling for what is causing his skin rash?"

She replied, "Yes, he breaks out from citric acid."

Wow! Impossible! I was never taught that citric acid causes eczema. Mary and I agreed to take all the citrus from Craig's diet to see if her incredible observation was possible, that citric acid caused his eczema. She came back to see me with Craig in two weeks. Incredibly, his skin was much clearer, perhaps a 50% improvement. She was right—citric acid was a cause of his eczema.

The remaining 50% bothered me, however, and I questioned Mary about any other causes she might have noticed but, unfortunately, she knew of no other cause.

I thought about Mary's observation about citrus, realizing it probably was a piece of the jigsaw puzzle I was seeking, and combined it with what Joyce had taught me about her kitchen-cleanser bath. I could think of only one connection between these two events: eczema had been caused by sensitivity to citric acid! When Joyce or Craig ate or drank too much citrus, the excess citrus irritated the nerves of their skin, which caused the itching skin. Citric acid, in essence, burned their skin!

I realized that eczema can be thought of as an acid burn of the skin! And, if that was so, then that explained why Joyce's skin healed with the kitchen-cleanser bath. The cleanser, which was alkaline, neutralized and washed away the citric acid, allowing the skin to heal.

This experience alerted me to a monstrous problem: allergists were unaware that this food chemical made millions of miserable people itch and scratch. Further, if we were unaware of this food chemical sensitivity to citric acid, how many other troubling food sensitivities lurked undiagnosed in our patients?

I knew then there must be other hidden, allergy-related food chemicals because Craig, although improved by eliminating citrus, was still troubled by something. I suspected that that mysterious something was in his diet—another troublesome food chemical like citric acid.

This thought prompted my search for the other food chemicals that culminated in the discovery of the aging food chemicals that cause my patients' distress.

I wish I had known about these chemicals back when I was treating Craig. I would have immediately eliminated from his diet the other common, but exasperating, aging food chemicals. I believe Craig's skin rash would have relented and his torment would have subsided.

Telling you that story allows me to introduce into our discussion a number of concepts, including: sensitivity to citric acid; the skin condition eczema; and the treatment of eczema.

Defining Citric Acid, Eczema, and Atopic Dermatitis

Citric acid

Citric acid is a natural, weak organic acid that is found in many fruits and vegetables, especially the citrus fruits. These citrus fruits are many and they are particularly rich in citric acid. A few of them are popular in our modern diet: oranges, lemons, limes and grapefruit. Pineapple and grapes also contains citric acid in appreciable quantities.

Our bodies naturally contain large quantities of citric acid and we use it for several purposes including producing energy and building protein. The body tolerates this natural content of citric acid, which does not precipitate the symptoms associated with citric acid sensitivity. However, when sensitive people eat and/or drink excess citric acid it does precipitate symptoms.

The large amount of citric acid in the modern diet is new; citric acid was isolated and identified less than one thousand years ago, so it has not been a part of our diet long enough for us to be genetically programmed to handle it. To restate this: in people sensitive to citric acid, the genes and the switches that control these genes have not had the many thousands of years necessary to acquire the gene modifications that would handle the amount of citric acid many of us consume.

This excess acid irritates our skin, making it itch. Based on my decades of research with my patients, it is my assertion that this happens because the high concentration of acid is filtered into our sweat glands, from which it emerges through our perspiration onto the skin where it burns the skin, creating the itchy rash known as eczema.

Eczema

"Eczema," itself, is a nonspecific term for many types of skin inflammation. The eczema we have been discussing is specifically atopic dermatitis, a long-lasting, chronic skin rash that causes intense skin itching. It is important to note that the term atopic comes from "atopy," which means "associated with or caused by allergy." In some eczema sufferers, a food or inhalant allergy aggravates the rash. Further suggesting allergy, other allergic symptoms such as hay fever and allergic asthma often accompany atopic dermatitis. However, in my allergy practice, sensitivity to citric acid was a more potent cause of the rash than was a true allergy.

In infancy, eczema or atopic dermatitis appears mainly on the face and scalp (probably from a combination of the citric acid found in mother's milk and from the mechanical rubbing of the face against the sheets) and often in the diaper area (most likely from citric acid in the stool). The associated rash can be so severe it can result in blisters that ooze and crust over. In adults, the rash appears as red to off-red patches that at times have small raised bumps that leak fluid—in severe cases, scratching brings a crusty, itching rawness to the skin.

The rash from eczema can appear all over the body, or it can concentrate at the ankles and wrists. Characteristic sites of involvement are at the bends of the elbow and behind the knees (this may be because these areas have softer, more irritation-prone skin that perspires more—lending credibility to the theory of citric acid coming through the sweat glands). It also occurs on the hands—resulting in what is often called dishwasher's hands (a combination of dryness of the hands involved with cleansing clothes and dishes and sensitivity to citric acid).

This rash needs to be differentiated from the rash resulting from contact dermatitis, which can also be red, raw, and itchy. Contact dermatitis usually begins with tiny—almost impossible to see—fluid-filled swellings of the skin appearing quickly (in minutes) or slowly (hours) after touching whatever is causing the contact dermatitis. Severe contact dermatitis irritates, itches, and hurts much more than the itch from severe atopic dermatitis. (For reference, a common cause of contact dermatitis is the oil from the poison ivy plant.)

The Impact of Eczema/Atopic Dermatitis

The number of people afflicted by eczema makes it a significant problem. A substantial portion of the US population has symptoms of eczema.

Eczema in Infants and Children.

That adults are affected by citric acid sensitivity is no surprise as aging most probably has the same weakening effect on the body's handling of citric acid as it does on the handling of MSG. However, it is surprising that many infants and young children are also affected. After all, they are not old and their genes have not aged and weakened.

I believe the best explanation for this sensitivity in the young is that atopic dermatitis is caused by many factors, including genetic predisposition, that make people susceptible to the itch and rash of citric acid. (And this genetic predisposition has been found in some rare cases of atopic dermatitis.) Whatever the cause, the treatment includes reducing the amount of citric acid in the diet of the young to the amount they are able to tolerate.

Eczema in Adults

Atopic dermatitis can also start in adults and this late-onset eczema aligns with the concept that aging genes can no longer metabolize a large amount of citric acid in our diets. Traditional treatment, sometimes, can be of limited help.

The traditional treatment of eczema includes using a mild soap to avoid drying out the skin, and a moisturizer to conserve the body's natural moisture immediately after a bath. For years, doctors treating adults suffering from eczema have told them to take warm, short showers (because hot, long showers dry out the skin); to reduce any stress that may make the itchiness worse; and to use medicines such as over-the-counter topical hydrocortisone and antihistamines for mild eczema. At times, adult sufferers of severe eczema have been treated with oral cortisone, ultraviolet light treatment, immunosuppressant/immunomodulator drugs and prescription-strength cortisone lotions.

For eczema prevention, the following treatments have been advised both by medical doctors and lay practitioners: using moisturizers daily and within three minutes of bathing or showering, after lightly patting your skin dry; using a humidifier; wearing soft clothing; avoiding temperature changes and sweating; and keeping fingernails short to reduce harm caused by scratching; and even recommendations to consider removing carpeting from living spaces and treating pets for dander.

In all these suggestions, there is no mention of using the treatment Joyce and Craig taught me: reducing the amount of citric acid in the diet. Sometimes, out of frustration, I yearn to shake the doctors treating patients with eczema and say, "Instead of all these actions to relieve and prevent the itch, tell your patients to reduce the amount of irritating acids reaching their skin. Try citric acid avoidance; it's safe and in many of your eczema patients, it will help!"

Other Symptoms of Citric Acid Sensitivity

One peculiar—but very common—symptom of citric acid sensitivity is cold sores or fever blisters. They are small but annoying fluid-filled blisters, usually around the lips and in the mouth, that break easily, discharging their watery fluid and then forming a crust as they heal. Let me be clear that citric acid does not cause these cold sores (blame a herpes virus that made a home in the nerves that control and protect the lips and mouth—activation of the herpes virus causes the cold sores). However, in many citrus-sensitive people I have found that citric acid powerfully irritates these virus-damaged nerves, proving it has the same power to damage nerves that is found in the other aging food chemicals.

Eating and drinking more citric acid than a person tolerates worsens all the distress associated with the cold sores, including increasing their frequency, their size, the discomfort they cause, and their duration. It also increases the number of cold sores that appear with each episode. I know all of this because all of these complications affect many of my patients—and they also affect me. If I have too much citric acid, I will soon develop one or more large, annoying cold sores on my lips or on the roof of my mouth.

I remember very well a patient who suffered many years of cold sores, each involving a crop of sores, appearing in many areas all over his mouth and lips. He was shocked to hear that citric acid may be responsible for making the cold sores so miserable—and equally shocked when avoiding citric acid dramatically reduced the impact of these miserable sores.

A Teachable Moment: A Mouth Swelling

One further event helped me understand the potency of citric acid in injuring nerves. I had convinced myself that I could tolerate the amount of acid in table grapes and ate them every morning for breakfast. After several weeks of indulging in these little balls of taste, the entire roof of my mouth swelled up. Upon reflection, I realized that the most likely explanation for the swelling was that the acids in the grapes damaged the nerves that typically maintained the integrity of the roof of my mouth. As they were not able to continue protecting the mouth, the roof of my mouth swelled. After I stopped eating grapes, the swelling lasted three weeks and then subsided, leaving no lasting damage. Even so, it left me with a good lesson in the ability of citric acid to irritate and damage nerves.

This episode, although uncomfortable, led me to the following conclusions: as a known sufferer from the effects of the aging chemicals, I cannot tolerate excess acid from grapes. As it is a sensitivity, instead of an allergy, I can still eat grapes but only in amounts that do not stress my tolerance. The episode reinforced the concept that citric acid, in excess, is a nerve toxin. My recovery showed me that nerves can return to normal function by avoiding the food that caused the irritation. This is important: damaged nerves can recover!

Where Citric Acid Is Found

As I mentioned at the start of this section, citric acid is found, of course, in the citrus fruits—oranges, lemons, limes, and grapefruit—with lemons containing the largest amount of citric acid in this group. You can certainly exceed your tolerance for citric acid by drinking orange juice and lemonade and eating oranges. If you notice your symptoms worsening, limit your intake of these foods. You can also exceed your tolerance by drinking citrus-flavored drinks, which you can identify by their fruity taste and by reading the list of ingredients. Citric acid—

known for adding "brightness" to many food flavor profiles—is often used in Mediterranean and Far Eastern dishes, and as a sort of condiment in many fish dishes, so you must be cautious and pay attention to your food intake if you are concerned about citric acid sensitivity.

Are Other Acids Involved in Citric Acid Sensitivity?

Other acids with similarities to citric acid are malic acid, tartaric acid, fumaric acid, and succinic acid. Because these have many of the same traits as citric acid, let us look at them, here.

Malic Acid

Like citric acid, malic acid is formed in the cells of our bodies and present in the foods we eat. Also like citric acid, it participates in the formation of protein and is a flavor enhancer (while citric acid gives foods a pronounced sour taste, malic acid's contribution is a milder sourness which persists longer than the sour taste of citric acid). Like the glutamic acid in MSG, these acids intensify the flavors in food and beverages by directly stimulating the nerves in the taste buds. As I have mentioned, a food chemical that causes nerve stimulation to taste buds can also cause muscle, organ, and other nerve stimulation and irritation—or even nerve destruction.

People sensitive to citric acid should use malic acid carefully, avoiding the excess that causes atopic dermatitis, cold sores, and mouth swelling. The amount of malic acid produced and used in the body is not a danger; the body can handle the acids that it produces and uses daily. And we can ignore the "usual" dietary levels of malic acid, since its level in food and beverages is typically low and sensitive people tolerate small amounts of this acid, just as they tolerate limited amounts of the other aging food chemicals. Only when a person's diet includes excess food chemicals like citric or malic acid will the body suffer.

I was never able to gauge the degree of harm caused by malic acid because, once my patients learned that their symptoms were caused by food chemicals, they stopped eating and drinking excessive amounts of the candies, gum, desserts, bakery products, and other processed foods and diet soft drinks that contained excess malic acid. If they returned to eating and drinking these foods and beverages, the painful headaches, annoying sleeplessness, and/or cramping abdominal pain returned, which reinforced their devotion to avoiding these troubling food chemicals.

Fumaric Acid

The story is the same with fumaric acid, which is the most sour of the food acids, as for citric and malic acid: the amount produced and used daily in the body is handled well. I believe it possesses the same nerve-injury power as citric and glutamic acid, but fewer people suffer from sensitivity to it because there is far less of it in the diet for sensitive people to eat and drink.

Succinic Acid

Succinic acid is another relative of this group of acids. It seems to be growing in popularity for a range of homeopathic uses as its synthesis becomes easier. My patients had limited exposure to it, however.

Tartaric Acid

Tartaric acid is an acid that is not found in large quantities in the body but found in many plants, especially grapes—and in the wine made from grapes. Wine makes some people feel sick and its content of tartaric acid may be a reason for this distress (I have already told you about my own reaction to grapes). In the average diet it is used as another of the sour flavor enhancers. Sensitive people should limit their consumption of wine if they tolerate tartaric acid poorly.

To summarize my feeling about excess consumption of these food acids: I fear them. I believe they have great potential for harm.

In many of my patients, citric acid worsens or causes many cases of atopic dermatitis, probably through direct irritation of the nerve fibers to the skin that make the skin itch.

Medical science knows that chronic herpes virus infection of the facial nerves causes cold sores and I found that citric acid significantly worsens these cold sores. It is also known from various studies that the chickenpox virus, herpes zoster, chronically infects the nerves of the body. Reactivation of this virus causes the severely itchy/painful skin rash called shingles, which typically appears on the face or body, and is most likely worsened by the citric acid we eat and drink.

Studies indicate that herpes and other viruses can also invade and chronically infect the nerves of the brain itself (part of the central nervous system). In a person made sensitive by chronic brain infection, a diet with excess citric acid may precipitate the same nerve damage to brain tissue which can be seen in flagrant cold sores, shingles, severe atopic dermatitis, and the swelling of the mouth I experienced. I believe that if the consumption of excess citric acid is stopped in time, healing can be complete. However, if excess consumption of citric acid is continued in people with chronic nerve/brain infections, damage may become permanent, and mental ability may be permanently lost.

Remember, if you are sensitive to citric acid, this does not mean you must completely avoid this (or other) food acids. To prevent or recover from the nerve damage they cause, just limit the amount you consume to the amount you tolerate.

Citric Acid Sensitivity and Nerves: A Summary

In this chapter and in previous chapters, we have discussed some characteristics of the aging food chemicals. I described how each of them has the potential to injure nerves. This is the case with the food acids mentioned here. Some of the damage caused by excess citric acid is readily apparent: rashes, mouth swelling, and cold sores. Some damage may be hidden, and may include the damage and/or destruction of the central nervous system and the mental deterioration and memory loss all of us fear. In short, you should be very alert for any signs that these acids hurt you, and act accordingly.

Chapter 8

Lactose—the Gassy Food Chemical

Lactose is a sugar, but it is not a "refined sugar," it comes from breast or cow's milk. Lactose is important at this point in our discussion because, first, it has been intensively studied—more than any other of the aging chemicals. (Fortunately, we can apply much of the knowledge gained from the study of lactose to the food chemicals we already examined.) Second, the role lactose plays in nerve injury and destruction is not as clear as the role of the other food chemicals, though I believe that it may be a cause of nerve damage.

Lactose differs from the other food chemicals we have discussed in several key ways: scientists have discovered the cause of lactose sensitivity; researchers have performed creditable peer-reviewed clinical studies; and doctors have developed evidence-based methods of treatment.

Why Lactose Must Be Included in the Group of Aging Food Chemicals

With the above differences, and acknowledging the uncertainty of its power to harm nerves, lactose still must be included in this discussion because, in my multitude of patients suffering from these aging chemicals, lactose sensitivity was almost always present. If patients denied sensitivity to lactose, and offered convincing proof they were not sensitive (such as being able to drink without symptoms more that one glass of cow's milk each day), I doubted that they suffered from the effects of the aging chemicals. But—almost always—they failed to provide this proof. In fact, I cannot remember a food chemical-sensitive patient who was not also sensitive to lactose. Therefore, lactose has joined the other chemicals as either a cause of nerve damage or an innocent bystander linked to them like each link of a chain connects to the next.

My patients, who were lactose sensitive but denied this sensitivity, were not lying when they denied their sensitivity to the lactose in cow's milk. They equated lactose sensitivity with milk allergy. But, lactose sensitivity is not an allergy. After all, with a food allergy even a small amount of milk can cause quickly appearing hives, tongue swelling, or other uncomfortable and even dangerous symptoms. As we know, food sensitivity often arises slowly—even sluggishly—hours after a meal, and only occurs when the sensitive person eats or drinks more of the specific food or beverage than can be tolerated.

When my patients denied being lactose sensitive, I became anxious that I was considering the wrong diagnosis. My anxiety over the missing lactose sensitivity would usually evaporate when I asked: "How much milk do you drink in a day?" When they answered, "Only enough for cereal in the morning," I knew my patients had limited tolerance for lactose, making it more likely they were also sensitive to the other aging chemicals.

My typical lactose-sensitive patients can tolerate small amounts of milk without symptoms; they can drink four ounces of lactose-containing milk each day. If they told me that they drank more than four ounces I then asked if they suffered from intestinal gas. If the answer was "yes," I knew lactose was giving them the gas and I could be comfortable with the diagnosis. If the answer was "no," I became very uncomfortable with the diagnosis of both lactose sensitivity and sensitivity to the aging chemicals and started looking for another diagnosis. (It turns out that my patients were often unaware of the difference between a food sensitivity and a food allergy and, when they denied sensitivity to milk, were really saying that they were not allergic to milk.)

Why Do Patients Deny the Cause of Their Condition?

As a doctor, I found that patients are typically smart and observant, possessing great "street smarts." Subconsciously, most of them knew—before they came to me for evaluation—which foods were causing their discomfort. However, they had trouble admitting it to themselves.

I learned that my task was to elevate awareness of their sensitivity from their subconscious minds, where it lay hidden, to their conscious minds—where they could acknowledge their sensitivity and deal with it. I could see in their faces the struggle to avoid accepting this diagnosis. I needed sympathy and kindness to help them achieve their realizations.

If my diagnosis was right, I could follow the play of emotion across their faces that transitioned from "No! That cannot be right!" to "OMG, it is right!" Then came the smile that said, "All right, I have been hiding it from myself." These words, although apparent in their facial expressions, were almost never spoken to me.

Some patients, however, simply could not admit—even to themselves—that the foods they craved made them suffer. They told me flat-out, "I cannot accept that diagnosis." I thanked them for their honesty, wished I had the tests that would tell them that my diagnosis was right, and wished them good luck in finding a diagnosis and treatment that would give them relief. Typically, I could refer them to no other doctor because their primary doctor—and then perhaps a gastroenterologist or neurologist—had already referred them to me because the appropriate tests showed no diagnosis.

After about two years of living in denial, many of these patients returned to me and told me they had finally followed my dietary advice and brought their symptoms under control. These follow-up visits made me feel very happy—yet sad that these people had wasted so much of their time being unhappy and feeling ill.

You may wonder why I am able to specify that they returned "after about two years." I can specify this because so many patients in my practice reacted to the aging food chemicals that the "some" who refused the diagnosis became a large number. I noticed that it invariably took this group about two years of suffering before they would accept the diagnosis and return to me to seek the care that brought them relief.

I have mentioned this group of patients because I want to stress that reversing your mental deterioration or restoring feeling to your feet and legs means you very well may need to limit your intake of foods you love to eat. Please understand—because it affects so many people—if you suffer symptoms that might be caused by these food chemicals, they probably are caused by them. I want to warn you: do not deny the possibility that you might also have to change your diet. Instead, you should embrace the possibilities, change your diet, and see if you can bring your symptoms under control.

Not All Lactose Sensitivity Is the Same

Several conditions can cause patients to suffer temporary lactose sensitivity, including viral infection of the intestine; inflammation of the intestine from Crohn's disease; irritable bowel syndrome; or major trauma to the intestines (including abdominal surgery). Although these conditions—as well as age or genes—can cause sensitivity to lactose, these temporary lactose sensitivities are not the subject of this book. We are discussing lactose sensitivity that is not temporary. The sensitivity we are discussing is permanent and much of it is caused by age and your genetic makeup.

We are also not discussing certain types of lactose sensitivity that are permanent, including the type that affects patients with celiac disease and another that severely affects infants who are unable to digest lactose. Further, we are not discussing galactosemia, a condition in which people are sensitive to the galactose sugar in milk. Patients suffering from any of the above issues must follow the advice of their family doctors, internists, pediatricians, or gastroenterologists—not the advice in this book.

The Genetics of Lactose Sensitivity

The lactose sensitivity we are discussing—late-onset and not complicated by any of the above conditions—is the common lactose sensitivity that afflicts millions. Studies have identified the cause as changes in a gene—LCT—that allow us to absorb and use lactose. The LCT gene instructs cells to make the enzyme lactase, which splits lactose. The human intestinal tract cannot absorb lactose until the two sugars that make up the lactose molecule, glucose and galactose, are split apart by the lactase. This lactase enzyme acts like a tiny man who pounds a wedge between the two sugar molecules of lactose, forcing them apart so they can be digested separately.

As most of us age, another gene, MCM6, progressively slows LCT's action. It acts like a switch that throttles down LCT's power to digest lactose, significantly lowering our ability to absorb and use lactose. This weakening of our ability for lactose digestion is why my lactose-sensitive patients can only drink about four ounces of lactose-containing milk each day without symptoms.

It is easy to see why babies need the lactase enzyme to absorb and use large amounts of lactose-containing milk. If they lose the source of mother's milk (from the death of the mother or her inability to produce breast milk), they could become severely malnourished or they could even die if they could not use a human breast milk substitute such as lactose-containing cow's milk.

Races of people who have raised cattle and drunk cow's milk as adults for thousands of years—for example, people of northern European backgrounds—commonly retain the ability to digest lactose. This continued ability to use cow's milk occurs because of mutations in the genes that allow the consumption and metabolism of lactose in adults. However, people whose ancestors as adults did not drink cow's milk —for example, people of African, Asian, Arab, Jewish, Greek, Italian, Hispanic, and American Indian backgrounds— commonly, as adults, lose much of their ability to digest lactose.

What Lactose Sensitivity Teaches Us about the Sensitivity to the Aging Chemicals

My experience with gluten-sensitive patients showed me that lactose sensitivity is attached to the aging chemicals like a hand is attached to a wrist. My experience also taught me that lactose sensitivity usually precedes sensitivity to the other food chemicals, including gluten, MSG, refined sugar, citric acid, and low-calorie sweeteners. If the syndrome were a marching band, lactose would be in front swinging the baton.

The Symptoms of Lactose Sensitivity

The six food chemicals share some symptoms such as tiredness, and simply not feeling well; each also has symptoms specific to the individual food chemical. Lactose intolerance also has its own symptoms, caused by undigested lactose in the intestines leading to the buildup of gas. The gas forms because, as we age, the lactase enzyme that breaks apart the two sugars of lactose can no longer handle a large load of lactose. The undigested lactose then passes through the intestine to the last part of the intestine, the large intestine.

In the large intestine, lactose meets live bacteria fully capable of digesting it. Unfortunately, the bacterial digestion produces large volumes of gas and irritates the intestine. Within thirty minutes to two hours after drinking too much milk, people with lactose sensitivity can suffer stomach cramps and diarrhea. These two symptoms point to the diagnosis of lactose sensitivity. And the presence of abdominal cramping suggests that the digestion of lactose by bacteria in the large intestine stimulates the nerves that cause abdominal cramping.

The associated gas production is no slight problem. It can be voluminous and smelly. I know because I am lactose sensitive and it is no fun evaluating patients while suffering this symptom in a small exam room. I am embarrassed to confess this symptom to you but I feel I must. I want you to remember that I suffer from sensitivity to these aging food chemicals, including lactose sensitivity, giving me a unique insight into the syndrome, increasing my ability to describe it to you, and making me more determined to tell you about it.

Treatment of Lactose Sensitivity (Lactase Deficiency)

I consider milk, with its content of calcium, important in the diet. Nature does, too. Modern studies point strongly to the beneficial effects of milk: adults able to drink milk are healthier and therefore better able to have descendants to pass on these beneficial lactose-tolerant genes. Over thousands of years, this has resulted in certain races with large numbers of members who, as adults, are tolerant of lactose.

However, some recent studies indicate that, as an adult, drinking cow's milk may not be healthy. (Further studies should eventually confirm or deny this possibility.) At the same time, any super-pasteurized milk can have too much MSG for many people because of the breakdown of milk proteins during pasteurization. Further, although there are milk substitutes, including soy milk, yogurt, and cheese, they contain—or may contain—high quantities of MSG imparted to the milk during processing.

There are certain steps you can take if you must limit your intake of lactose-containing milk:

1) First, consult with your doctor and/or dietician.

2) Peruse the information available on the Internet.

3) Drink daily as much lactose-containing milk as you can tolerate without symptoms and/or drink lactose-free cows' milk if you tolerate it. (See above note on MSG.)

4) Supplement your diet with calcium if advised by your doctor or dietician.

5) Eat calcium-containing foods (dark, leafy greens like spinach, kale, turnips greens, or collard greens).

What Treating Hundreds of Lactose Sensitive/ Intolerant Patients Taught Me

I am grateful for the many lactose-sensitive patients whose insight into their condition taught me much about lactose sensitivity and its relation to the aging chemicals including:

- The coexistence of lactose sensitivity and sensitivity to the other aging chemicals in so many patients indicates that they belong to the same group of problem-causing chemicals.

- Stimulation of the nerves causing cramps and diarrhea suggests that lactose causes nerve irritation. Nerve irritation is a characteristic of the aging chemicals.

- Weakened or dimmed genes cause lactose sensitivity.

- The increased incidence of lactose intolerance in the population as it ages is compatible with the concept that aging is a cause of sensitivity to lactose and to the other aging food chemicals.

- These sensitivities are not an illness or sickness, they are a normal consequence of aging—even the aging of an infant into a child.

- The sensitivities arise from the decreasing ability of the body's workhorses—enzymes—to digest these chemicals.

- Our modern diet overflows with these aging chemicals, an

96

overflow that started recently, from a genetic standpoint.

❧ Because the aging chemicals taste good, we often eat them in excess.

❧ The desire for these chemicals makes the sufferer ignore the symptoms caused by their presence.

❧ Because they were tolerated well in early life, the contribution of these food chemicals to distressing symptoms often hides from the afflicted sufferer.

Chapter 9

The Aging Food Chemicals and Nerve-related Illnesses

So far I have concentrated on the adverse effects of eating or drinking MSG, low-calorie sweeteners, gluten, refined sugar, citric acid, and lactose. I showed you that these chemicals (with the possible exception of lactose) are neurotoxins. Why should that worry you?

You should worry because neurotoxins we consume in our diet can worsen the impact of such ailments as:

- Alzheimer's disease,
- Mild cognitive impairment,
- Parkinson's disease,
- Huntington's Chorea,
- Multiple sclerosis,
- Amyotrophic lateral sclerosis,
- Diabetic neuropathy,
- Stroke, and
- Migraine headaches.

To put it simply: a person suffering a disease caused by damaged and dying nerves should not consume neurotoxins.

Now that you know more about the aging food chemicals, you can see why I refer to them as "aging." As we grow older, the genes that protect us from these food chemicals also grow older; they slow down, dim, and lose much of their protective power. If we do not lower the amount of these chemicals that we consume they can injure and destroy the nerves that control thinking, memory, balance, and so many of our basic bodily functions—the same deterioration we see in an aging person.

In this chapter our discussion will concentrate on illnesses or diseases related to nerve damage and destruction. In these conditions, the average person's diet can actually promote the truly horrendous deterioration that characterizes these malicious diseases. And I do mean "malicious"; what else would you call a disease that damages the brain?

1. Alzheimer's disease

We start with Alzheimer's disease because of my personal experience with mental deterioration—the same deterioration experienced by sufferers of this disease. In this disease the aging chemicals can destroy the nerves essential to our thoughts and memories. They can, and do, change an independent and useful member of society into a baby-like dependent. They destroy their victim's freedom.

The National Institute on Aging identifies early symptoms of Alzheimer's as including memory loss, getting lost, taking longer at normal daily tasks, and experiencing difficulty with speaking, reading, writing, and adding and subtracting numbers (Alzheimer's Disease Fact Sheet, 2015). I have personally discovered that these symptoms affect me whenever I indulge in the aging food chemicals.

The Alzheimer's Association lists ten warning signs of Alzheimer's, and the sixth sign is: "New problems with words in speaking or writing." They go on to say that: "People with Alzheimer's may have trouble following or joining a conversation. They may stop in the middle of a conversation and have no idea how to continue or they may repeat themselves. They may struggle with vocabulary, have problems finding the right word or call things by the wrong name (e.g., calling a "watch" a "hand-clock") (10 Early Signs and Symptoms of Alzheimer's, 2016).

My experience with trying to give a simple introduction to a speaker is a good illustration of the above points. I had exceeded my tolerance of the aging chemicals for far too long and my speech became halting and I could not finish sentences.

Prevention/Treatment of Alzheimer's Disease

I often think of a simple story that points to the treatment of Alzheimer's-related mental deterioration:

Four men bought new houses with wooden siding and each painted his house, the first man with expensive and strongly protective paint, the second, third, and fourth with progressively cheaper paints. To keep their houses scrupulously clean, each—once or twice daily—sprayed the house with an acid bath. The first house, painted with the best paint, showed no damage from the spray after eighty years. After fifty years, the less-protecting paint on the second house showed mild paint pitting and loss of luster from the acid spray. The third house, with even less protective paint, showed more severe damage and the fourth house—with the cheapest paint—suffered such damage from the spray that it was completely uninhabitable.

In this story, we are the houses; the acid sprays are the neurotoxins we eat daily; and the paints protecting the homes are the genes that protect us from these diet chemicals. Some of us are lucky and, like the first home, we are protected by our genes that act like the expensive paint; they allow us to safely eat the sugar and neurotoxins that harm others until we reach old age. Some of us are like the homes protected by the less-expensive paints, our genes only partially protect us; they allow mental decline to appear at about forty to sixty years of age. Some of us are like the house that was completely devastated by the acid washes. Incompetent genes fail us so completely that we suffer harm from our diet at an even younger age.

You may be asking yourself: "Why do those homeowners use an acid spray to clean their homes?" It is because they do not realize how much harm the spray can cause. We eat refined sugar, low-calorie sweeteners, citric acid, and neurotoxins like MSG for the same reason: we do not realize (or acknowledge) the harm these chemicals can cause.

How do our homeowners stop the deterioration of their homes? They stop spraying them with acid washes. How do we stop (or slow) the deterioration of our minds? We stop eating and drinking foods and beverages with excessive levels of aging food chemicals.

Is it silly to use an example where owners spray their homes with acids? Yes! They should never have started. Is it silly for us to eat and drink foods containing neurotoxins? Yes! We should never have started.

Why We Are Sensitive to the Aging Chemicals

On the most basic level, we are sensitive to these chemicals because we live too long. For countless eons, our non-human and then human ancestors died early of disease or starvation—or due to attacks by predators. Because life was so short, only a few of us developed the genes that, as we grow older, detoxify the large amount of neurotoxins in our diets that are so well tolerated by the young.

With injury to—and death of—nerve cells characterizing Alzheimer's disease, to prevent further deterioration and reverse the deterioration already present, we must feed Alzheimer's disease sufferers a diet that contains only as much of the aging chemicals as they can tolerate without further nerve damage.

2. Mild Cognitive Impairment

People with mild cognitive impairment (MCI) suffer memory or other thought-related problems but are not as disabled as those people suffering with Alzheimer's disease. Unfortunately, as they age, more of these people progress to Alzheimer's disease compared with those without mild cognitive impairment.

Prevention/Treatment of Mild Cognitive Impairment

Studies show a relationship between diabetes and mild cognitive impairment. Refined sugar is a cause—or aggravating factor—in diabetes, and people suffering this disorder should more stringently avoid refined sugar as they avoid other neurotoxins. After all, it makes no sense to feed people with mild cognitive impairment foods and beverages containing increased amounts of the aging chemicals.

3. Parkinson's Disease

This disease occurs due to the death of certain cells in the brain that produce a chemical called dopamine. Dopamine is a neurotransmitter—as is glutamic acid—by which nerve cells send signals to other nerve cells. With the decrease in dopamine, muscle activity is affected, resulting in shaking, rigidity, slowness of movement, and difficulty with walking and keeping an even gait. Often, cognitive and behavioral problems can occur, which can progress, in advanced stages, to dementia.

Prevention/Treatment of Parkinson's Disease

Genetic causes are known in a subset of Parkinson's disease sufferers and are suspected in many more. However, whether Parkinson's disease is caused by a known genetic cause or not, because nerve cell injury and death characterize this disease, I believe it makes no sense to feed people with Parkinson's disease foods and beverages with excess aging food chemicals.

4. Huntington's Disease

Huntington's disease (formerly known as Huntington's chorea) is a genetic disorder that involves the death of nerve cells throughout the brain—but most prominently in the area of the brain called the basal ganglia; these cells play a key role in movement and behavior control. The term "chorea" actually refers to a disorder involving brief, repetitive, jerky, involuntary movement. As this disease progresses, the sufferer's cognitive abilities are progressively diminished.

Prevention/Treatment of Huntington's Chorea
Because it is best to limit our self-inflicted destruction of nerve cells, it is best to avoid excess aging food chemicals.

5. Multiple Sclerosis
Multiple sclerosis (MS) is a disease caused by the body's own immune system attacking the central nervous system (which includes the brain, spinal cord, and optic nerves). The primary attack is directed against myelin, the protective fatty/protein coat wrapping around the nerves' axons ("axons" are the projections from the nerves that reach to other nerve cells).

Through its effect on nerves, MS can impact almost every system of the body, triggering issues with eyesight, muscles, sensation, and the autonomic nervous system (damage to the autonomic nervous system can cause urinary incontinence, constipation, erectile dysfunction, vaginal dryness, hypotension, irregular heartbeat, and other symptoms). Where the MS damages the nervous system determines what symptoms will be experienced.

Prevention/Treatment of Muscular Sclerosis
Because the disease is characterized by nerve cell injury and nerve death, sufferers with multiple sclerosis should avoid foods with excess aging food chemicals.

6. Amyotrophic Lateral Sclerosis
The progressive destruction in the brain and spinal cord of the nerves that control muscle action can eventually lead to total paralysis in

amyotrophic lateral sclerosis (also known as "ALS" or "Lou Gehrig's disease"). The inherited form of this disease arises from mutated genes, although other genes may also be involved. One theory states that most likely the immune system participates in the destruction of these nerves, as does the mishandling of protein in nerve cells.

Prevention/Treatment of Amyotrophic Lateral Sclerosis

Most sufferers have higher levels of the neurotoxin glutamic acid (MSG) in the spinal fluid around the nerve cells. If you recall our discussion of MSG, you can understand why, with nerve cell impairment characterizing this disease, sufferers should avoid excess of the aging chemicals.

7. Diabetic Neuropathy

Alzheimer's Disease and Diabetes

There is evidence that Alzheimer's disease is a type of diabetes although, until the past few years most doctors recognized only two types of diabetes: type 1 and type 2. The relationship is complicated, though it is well discussed by the Alzheimer's Association in "Diabetes and Cognitive Decline" (2015).

Type 1 diabetes is also called "juvenile" or "insulin-dependent" diabetes, and usually starts before thirty years of age and affects a small but significant percentage of diabetics, who must take insulin daily. Type 2 or "non-insulin dependent" diabetes, affects 90 percent to 95 percent of the 26 million Americans with diabetes, who may or may not need to take insulin.

Complications of Diabetes

About half of the people with diabetes suffer from significant nerve injury. Any nerve can be affected, but the extremities are typically impacted; the legs and feet are most seriously affected. There, peripheral neuropathy (nerve damage) causes numbness and tingling in the feet and legs and can lead to muscle weakness and, ultimately, great pain in the arms and legs. Sufferers can be afflicted with a loss of feeling and the loss of the sensation that tells them (among other things) whether they are standing properly or falling over. The loss of this sensation causes tripping and falling, and the resultant bruising, broken bones, and further loss of sensation that can lead to amputation from unfelt and unnoticed injuries and infections.

This nerve damage also harms diabetics' blood vessels, hearts, gastrointestinal systems, and renal systems. Much of this damage is attributed to high levels of blood sugar.

Why Alzheimer's Disease Is Important to Diabetes

Today, throughout the world, about 35 million people suffer from Alzheimer's disease. As the population ages, by 2050 this number can be expected to rise to 100 million. In fact, the potential number of people with memory disorders is devastating. The cost of treating this epidemic is already overwhelming.

For years, medical scientists knew that type 2 diabetics were two to three times more likely to suffer Alzheimer's-related dementia than non-diabetics. The obese are similarly more likely to suffer Alzheimer's than the non-obese.

Obesity and insulin resistance are features of the aging food chemicals, especially the refined sugar that we already discussed. As we will see, the correlation between diabetes and Alzheimer's is strong, suggesting that diabetes predisposes its sufferers to Alzheimer's disease.

How Could the Aging Food Chemicals Cause Alzheimer's Disease?

If a person has the genetic ability to have diabetes—and that genetic ability is widespread as judged by the large numbers of diabetics—years of repeated consumption of the aging food chemicals can awaken a monster, the insulin resistance that characterizes diabetes. Combining refined-sugar-caused obesity and diabetes with dietary neurotoxin-caused nerve damage launches a dreadful one-two punch capable of causing or worsening the devastating effects of Alzheimer's disease.

As we discussed earlier, the body handles alcohol and fructose alike: both turn to fat in the liver and both can lead to the insulin insensitivity of diabetes. Both most likely harm the brain—alcohol through its direct effect on brain cells and its promotion of diabetes, fructose through its promotion of diabetes.

Prevention/Treatment of Diabetes
With nerve cell injury and nerve death characterizing this disease, persons suffering diabetic neuropathy should avoid foods containing excess of the aging food chemicals—especially refined sugar.

8. Migraine Headaches
As we discussed earlier, among my patients, the aging food chemicals are a major cause of painful migraine headaches.

Prevention/Treatment of Migraine Headaches
With nerve cell/artery irritation impacting those inflicted with migraines, headache sufferers should avoids foods and beverages with excess aging food chemicals.

Why Did I Keep Repeating the Above Prevention/ Treatment Advice?
Because the advice is the same in each condition, I hope repetition of this dietary avoidance plants this advice deeply in your mind so that you will not forget it.

A Clarification

Please be aware that I do not attribute the causes of all these diseases only to foods. I have tried to specify some of the other causes of these diseases—many known and many only suspected—including the involvement of our genes.

In fact, without the presence of the genes that permit these diseases, we would not suffer from many of them. But, once diseases begin, we must follow a treatment that can slow their progress.

As we have discussed, the foods that promote the progressive destruction of our nerves caused by these diseases are also the foods that activate our taste buds—in short, the foods that harm us also taste good. They also, unfortunately, activate, damage, and even kill nerves in our body and brain.

You Probably Cannot Change the Basic Course of Any Disease.

It may be cruel to say that you have no chance of changing your disease-prone fate, but it is also true. If your genes allow the diseases listed above, medical science cannot change your genes to free you from the fear of contracting any of those diseases. But there is hope. Although you and your medical caregiver cannot change the basic course of the disease, you can slow it down. The following is an explanation of how these diseases can be slowed.

You Probably Can Significantly Slow Down These Diseases

As an allergist, I have used injections to treat many patients for their allergies to house dust, mold, and pollen. It became apparent to me over the years that the injections had a wonderful affect on my patients' immune systems. As long as the injections contained house dust, they quieted the hyperactive immune system. Not only did the allergic symptoms caused by their immune systems quiet down—symptoms like severe hay fever and asthma—the shots also quieted symptoms of autoimmune diseases like lupus and multiple sclerosis.

Patients suffering autoimmune diseases like lupus and multiple sclerosis frequently suffer episodes where the disease flares into a heightened stage with increased symptoms, each seeming to leave the sufferer with progressive debility. I believe that these symptom spikes signal a significant activation of the autoimmune disease that accelerates the power of these diseases to harm. Stopping these spikes should—and in my patients did—slow the progression of the autoimmune disease. By reducing or eliminating these spikes, the injection treatment (which I was using for allergies) prevented the deterioration in the health of the patient which could have been caused by the spikes. Further, my patients' autoimmune disease did not seem to significantly worsen as long as the injection treatment continued. This is not to say that I would urge you to seek allergy injection treatments, but I wanted to give you an example of ways you can hinder the progression of autoimmune diseases in a safe way.

Connecting Autoimmune Diseases to Damaged Nerve Diseases

How much help can you expect from avoiding the aging food chemicals? As with the effect of the allergy injections on immune disease, you can expect significant help if you suffer a condition caused by deteriorating nerves, especially if you start avoiding these diet chemicals early in the course of your deterioration. Consider, again, my illustration of the four houses and their paint:

The house with the good paint had no deterioration, similar to the people who are not susceptible to nerve deterioration. They do not need to avoid these food chemicals.

The next two houses experienced deterioration from less-protective paint, similar to suffering nerve damage and nerve death. Avoiding the aging food chemicals can help you to fight against nerve deterioration much like stopping the acid wash helped to stop the house from deteriorating.

And, to make this treatment even more enticing I am convinced that we who suffer nerve deterioration can repair ourselves. We can regain the ability to remember, the ability to plan, the ability to tie our own shoes. We can live independently. The earlier we start the diet, the more complete the recovery can be. On the other hand, if we continue to feed ourselves the aging chemicals, the damage can become irreversible.

Remember that the last house was so damaged by the acid wash that it was not habitable. That house is like the patients on memory units in health care settings, who have been severely damaged. It is possible that, with careful dietary practices, we can avoid this outcome, and the progression of Alzheimer's disease, Lou Gehrig's disease, Parkinson's disease and other syndromes can be so altered that the progression of these severe states of debilitation can be prevented or delayed for many, many years. There is even a good chance that much of the damage can be reversed! We only need to try!

Chapter 10

Cautions and Notes about Avoiding the Aging Food Chemicals

We have discussed the aging chemicals separately. Now I want to discuss them as a group. I will review some of the information I already gave you and add some new information that I think will help you understand this food sensitivity and its treatment. I will also propose and answer some questions that probably bothered you as we discussed the aging food chemicals.

Who Needs to Avoid the Aging Chemicals?

Should Everyone Avoid the Foods and Beverages That Contain Excesses of the Aging Food Chemicals?

There are two answers to that question.

The First Answer

Yes, maybe everybody—even those free of the symptoms of nerve damage and destruction—should avoid these foods and beverages. Most likely, years of silent nerve destruction passes before the average sufferer notices nerve damage.

Even people with no symptoms or family history of nerve damage already may be suffering nerve damage.

This might be the right answer but I realize that it is not realistic. These food chemicals taste good and make meals tasty; without them a meal can taste flat. Therefore, if we are honest, we will have to admit that few people will avoid these foods and beverages if they are not threatened by the emergence of mental deterioration, the inability to feel their feet, or some other nerve disease.

The Second Answer

If you are noticing any symptoms of nerve damage or have a family history of Alzheimer's disease, Lou Gehrig's disease, diabetic loss of sensation in the legs and feet, or other diseases of nerve degeneration, you should certainly avoid these foods and beverages.

If you notice nerve damage in yourself or your loved ones, you should feel so threatened that you will take any available measures to fight off these tragic diseases. Medical caregivers may be able to tell you or a loved one that a genetic potential exists for nerve disease. If they do, and the tests indicate that you have a hereditary predisposition toward these diseases, avoiding these chemicals has great potential to prevent, or at least slow, nerve deterioration.

How Compulsively Must These Foods Be Avoided?

The answer, again, is two-fold:

If you or your loved one shows symptoms of nerve damage— especially mental deterioration—you (or your loved one) should compulsively avoid these foods, so that you can avoid hospitalization in the memory care units for advanced mental deterioration.

(I have visions of someday wandering through these memory care units and finding them empty. I believe this will happen and I believe that strict avoidance of the aging food chemicals will help empty these wards. That is why I wrote this book.)

The aging food chemicals are not harmful if consumed in small doses that people can tolerate. After all, they are vital constituents of the body. Prior to the time that symptoms appear, limited amounts of these chemicals can be consumed, apparently without harm, and especially in the young. However, as our age increases, and nerve damage in the brain or the extremities progresses, avoidance of the aging food chemicals must be more compulsive.

When we notice numbness and tingling of the extremities or increasing difficulty in remembering the events of the previous day, we must awaken to the realization that we are failing. Then we must reduce our intake of the chemicals that are destroying our nerves.

Wouldn't It Be Better to Start Compulsive Avoidance of Foods with Excesses of These Chemicals Early in Life?

Yes, absolutely. But, practically, how many of us will deny ourselves the wonderful luxury of an MSG-flavored steak or deny our children that delightful fructose-packed ice cream cone? Only when we become frightened enough for our future or that of a loved one will we completely change our diet.

How Long Does the Effect of Food Remain in the Body?

From my experiences and those of my patients, about three days. If, during a meal, you have consumed an unwise amount of the aging food chemicals, be especially careful to reduce your consumption of these chemicals in your food and beverages for at least three days to let your body heal.

Isn't This Avoidance Diet Too Difficult to Follow?

No, not at all when you consider its benefits.

You are undertaking a monumental task. Depending on your genetic makeup, your nerves may be injured and eventually destroyed if you, year after year, eat and drink foods and beverages that contain an excess of these neurotoxins, these aging chemicals.

You desperately want to stop the emergence or the progression of these symptoms. Even beyond that, you want to start reversing these symptoms—you want to think clearly; you want to feel your feet again; you want to slow down your shaking. These diet changes, along with lifestyle changes, should help you rebuild your nerves. Do not think of this avoidance as difficult, think of it as hopeful. Hopeful that, through avoiding these aging food chemicals you can continue to feel (or return to feeling) normal.

Can the Brain Recover Its Ability to Think and Plan, and the Peripheral Nerves Their Ability to Feel Sensations?

Doctors used to think that brain damage was irreversible. It is not! Both the brain and peripheral nerves can recover. One of the proofs of this recovery is found in the field of "face transplants." Nerves from the transplant grow into the underlying face and the brain learns to use these nerves.

Further, learning a new task or skill prompts the brain to expand the area involved in the activity. Therefore, we know that the brain can learn and adapt. If that can happen with face transplants and new learning, it can happen with you.

Is an Avoidance Diet Enough by Itself to Effectively Combat the Nerve Damage and Destruction That Leads to Mental Deterioration?

No. You need more than dietary avoidance. Our concentration in this book is on dietary chemicals you should avoid in your quest to slow or to prevent mental deterioration. Other measures such as physical and mental exercise are also important in repairing nerve destruction.

With these thoughts I end this portion of this book about the diet and how it may be causing your, or a loved one's, distressing nerve deterioration. As you try to avoid the foods I discussed, I hope that these diet changes will halt the progression of your debility. I further hope that—as in my early Alzheimer's disease experience—it guides you to a return of the health and youth that these food chemicals are trying to rob from you.

In the next section, we will look at both general and specific ways you can alter your diet as you pursue the good health that a proper diet brings.

PART 2

Food Planning and Preparation

Chapter 11
Planning Your Healthy Meals

We have examined how the food chemicals in the modern diet lead to multiple illnesses and disabilities, concentrating especially on the diet's power to cause mental deterioration. Now we will discuss how to apply what you have learned as you plan your daily meals. To determine how completely you need to clear your diet of these aging food chemicals, you first must determine how deeply these chemicals affect you.

There are millions of people who are sensitive to the aging diet chemicals and they suffer symptoms that can differ from those you suffer, and they can also differ in their degree of sensitivity. Because of this, how closely you and they need to follow the diet will also vary. You need to evaluate your own symptoms and degree of sensitivity to learn how closely you must follow the diet.

If your symptoms are mild, minor changes (such as stopping drinking diet soda pop or orange juice) may be all that is necessary. More severe symptoms such as repetitive migraine headaches or difficulty thinking or forming complete sentences should drive you to more comprehensive diet restrictions. If you are suffering symptoms that may force you into a memory unit, you must strictly follow the diet—beginning as soon as possible.

What Factors Influence the Severity of Your Symptoms?

Certainly age is a huge factor. Typically, as children, we suffered little from the aging food chemicals, because our genes had not yet weakened with age. As the years march on, our genes progressively weaken and our sensitivity to these chemicals strengthens, as do our symptoms and our need for caution in choosing our diet.

Another factor is the type of symptoms you are suffering. Repetitive, severe headaches should force you into following the diet closely. Trouble thinking and speaking should scare you as you contemplate a downhill course leading to an Alzheimer's-like dependent state. If you find yourself in this condition, you should follow the diet compulsively. Less frightening and milder symptoms will allow you to include a limited amount of these chemicals in your diet.

How Do You Know When You Have Exceeded Your Tolerance for the Food Chemicals?

You know when you have exceeded your tolerance for these food chemicals when your symptoms flare up. If, for instance, you suffer headaches or your headaches return or worsen; if you suffer poor sleep, your sleep is less restful, or you awaken too early; or if you suffer recurrent cold sores, they erupt, swell exasperatingly, and subside sluggishly.

You know you have exceeded your tolerance if you notice deterioration in your thinking or speaking, or numbness or shakiness. With any of these conditions, be sure to engage the help of medical caregivers. They can help you understand your condition and search for non-diet causes of your symptoms.

Now let us look at the foods that you can tolerate. You have much to gain by following this diet as it has significantly reversed the symptoms of aging in many people—including me. It could do the same for you. We will look at vitamins and alcoholic beverages, first, and then discuss a general approach to preparing and eating vegetables, fruits, and meats.

Taking Vitamins

Medical science is still trying to determine the benefits and disadvantages of vitamin supplements. I find I tolerate only limited amounts of vitamins, perhaps only one multivitamin infrequently instead of one daily. Even so, in northern winters, especially with older people, with limited exposure to the sun (such as the institutionalized), vitamin D may be worthwhile.

Alcoholic Beverages

The impact of alcohol on our nerves is a most difficult subject to summarize and I can only speculate on it. There is evidence both for and against the use of alcohol. The body handles alcohol as it handles fructose, by converting most of it into fat in the liver and encouraging the onset of the insulin resistance and peripheral neuropathy associated with diabetes. People sensitive to the aging food chemicals probably should either avoid alcohol, or drink very little of it.

Vegetables

I tolerate most fresh and frozen vegetables such as peas, beans, asparagus, and the cabbage family after I boil them for about five minutes and then discard the boiled water. I believe this boiling drives off any excess fructose and MSG content of the vegetables.

For a good vegetable protein source, I use beans boiled until soft.

I tolerate canned vegetables and other vegetable preparations if the list of ingredients does not contain the aging food chemicals.

Fruits

Farmers through the ages have extensively genetically altered many fruits, increasing their content of fructose—especially in apples, pears, berries, and grapes, as well as the wine made from grapes.

I fear the deleterious effect of citric acid on the brain so I avoid the citrus fruits, tomato preparations (remember: a tomato is a fruit), and fruit juices. I recommend that you limit their consumption and watch for signs of sleeplessness and itching.

Where the content of citric acid in what you are eating or drinking is low—possibly used only to preserve a food or drink, and not flavor it—it should be able to be tolerated.

Meats

In my allergy practice—even in patients either sensitive to or allergic to food—unprocessed meats including beef, pork, chicken, turkey, or fish are usually tolerated well. I also tolerate them well.

However, I avoid processed or manufactured meats if the aging food chemicals have been added. Food manufacturers often add MSG, "flavorings," sugar, and other troubling food chemicals to meat, all of which should be avoided.

Measure the Success of Your Diet Changes by Observing Your Quickly Appearing Symptoms

You can learn to track the severity of your symptoms in the same way I follow mine. I evaluate how well I am following my diet by the symptom control I am achieving. When I stray too far from the diet I note the following symptoms appearing within hours (or up to a day later).

My speech becomes seriously disrupted; I have trouble forming complete sentences.

Tasks that call for thinking, such as writing, become more difficult.

My ability for remembering numbers, names, dates, and appointments deteriorates significantly.

I experience diarrhea and constipation.

I can only sleep for a few hours before awakening.

My tear ducts itch uncomfortably. (The most likely cause of

the itch: the tear fluid from my eyes is trying to discharge the extra acid in my diet through my tear ducts. If I have even more acid, my skin itches—in the same way that a "skin itch" characterizes atopic dermatitis.)

You can evaluate the benefits of your diet by observing your own quickly appearing symptoms. They may be similar to the symptoms I experience or you may suffer other symptoms such as tiredness, headaches (including migraine or cluster headaches), or itchy rashes in the groin or rectal area. Remember that quickly appearing symptoms should subside after three days if you avoid consumption of the aging chemicals, since it takes about three days for any dietary chemical overload to leave the body.

Measure the Success of Your Diet Changes by Observing Your Chronic Symptoms

Chronic symptoms can include chronic headaches, chronic constipation, chronic itchy rashes, and chronic tiredness. They can also include the neurologic diseases we already discussed, such as Alzheimer's disease, ALS, and the others.

If you or a loved one suffer(s) from any of these diseases, and are sensitive to these aging chemicals, please remember that improvement with the diet may proceed slowly, taking months or even years to appear. After all, it took months (or years) of eating these food chemicals to develop your chronic symptoms, so you can't expect them to disappear overnight. You have to be patient and give symptom relief the time to show itself.

Be vigilant during this time to ensure that the aging chemicals are truly excluded from your diet. Also, understand that these chemicals, especially refined sugar, have addicting qualities, so eliminate foods and beverages containing excesses of these chemicals from your home so you are less tempted to eat (or drink) them for a snack.

Following the Diet—Initially

Initially, you should follow the diet strictly. If you remove all the foods containing excesses of the aging food chemicals from your diet you should gain pleasing relief of your symptoms. Initial symptom improvement may appear within days, assuming the condition that plagues you can be reversed in a few days. Even when initial relief appears within a few days, typically your symptoms will not entirely disappear but will continually improve over months (or years) until you gain the maximum relief the diet provides. Symptom improvement can continue as long as you are following the diet.

For instance, if your sensitivity to the aging chemicals—like mine—makes you forget words and suffer difficulty in forming sentences, you should notice better memory and sentence formation within days, and then continual speech improvement over months.

However, if you have suffered trouble thinking or memory loss for months or years, it may require months of strict avoidance of foods containing excess aging food chemicals before real relief begins. If the symptoms have lasted too long, and brain damage has progressed too far, there may be no improvement. However, even with long-time, distressing symptoms, you should not give up prematurely.

Why Does Improvement Take So Long?

I believe that injured nerves need time to become healthy, and damaged nerves need time to regrow. Your brain needs time to leave senility behind and your body needs time to regain its youth.

Now, with these thoughts about following the diet, let us look at what you can eat and drink. Remember, if you are allergic to any of the foods I suggest, do not eat them.

How I Follow the Diet

Breakfast

In the morning I try to eat a bowl of mixed berries such as blueberries or blackberries. I have to be careful not to exceed my tolerance to acidic foods and I stop eating the berries if I notice itchiness of my tear ducts.

I always eat a hearty breakfast including three eggs, sunny side up. Before placing the eggs in the frying pan I place a handful of walnut pieces in the pan and crack the eggs onto the walnut pieces so the fried eggs contain the walnut pieces.

Every other day I prepare and eat six slices of pan-fried bacon and, on the alternate day, I eat a meat patty I previously prepared and cooked.

I find it helpful to prepare a large amount of certain foods, such as meat patties, to use as part of my future meals. To prepare up to forty meat patties, I combine one pound each of ground pork and beef, as well as either chicken or turkey, by kneading them together with one cup each of chopped carrots, green pepper, and onion. I season to taste with rosemary, basil, and salt, then form the mixture into individual patties and bake at 350 degrees for thirty minutes or until the meat is cooked. (It's good to check the temperature of the meat with a meat thermometer.) Then I freeze the patties individually and use them to supplement my other meals (see below for a full recipe for these meat patties by Molly).

Daytime Snacks

If I am still hungry after breakfast I eat nuts, an apple, or a pear. However, because of their content of fructose, I limit my consumption of apples and pears to only one or the other each day. Nuts, including Brazil nuts, cashews, pistachios, and walnuts contain much glutamic acid, so I also limit them in my diet.

Celery and cauliflower are good snack foods, as are canned vegetables such as peas and green beans. If I am especially hungry between meals I will open a can of salmon and mix it with the vegetables above and eat until I am satisfied.

Noon Meal

My noon meal is always the same. As with breakfast, I use previously prepared food. To make this, I soak dried beans (black beans, garbanzo beans, soy beans, or other dried beans as desired) in water in a pot (filling only the bottom fourth of the pot to allow plenty of room for the swelling beans) for twenty-four hours, until the beans soften. I then drain and replace the water and boil the beans until they are soft.

After I drain the beans, I add about a cup each of peas, green beans, asparagus, frozen corn, and chopped carrots that I have boiled for five minutes. I mix the bean combination with the pea/carrot combination and put them into the freezer, re-mixing the combined preparation as it freezes to prevent it from turning into a block of ice. I make enough of this mixture to last several weeks. Then, as the supply dwindles, I again repeat the above process.

At the noon meal I pour the frozen vegetable combination into a bowl and often combine it with a bit of chopped fresh celery to add some crunch. I microwave this preparation on high for three minutes. This is then topped with fresh spinach and microwaved for an additional thirty seconds. Olive oil and other seasonings—without the aging food chemicals—can be added for flavor.

Evening Meal

The evening meal is the simplest. After a large breakfast and noon meal, I am only mildly hungry and content with a simple, small meal of chicken, turkey, beef, or pork sufficient for the meal, that I cook myself in a frying pan or pressure cooker. At times, the meat is accompanied by a salad of lettuce or cabbage tossed with carrots and onion, again using olive oil for the dressing.

Dessert

You've got to be kidding! The typical dessert has fructose as a sweetener. After losing eighty pounds by excluding fructose from my diet, I have no desire to return to eating it and regaining the weight.

Chapter 12

Tips from Molly Behymer of Creative Catering by Molly LLC

In the following section, Molly Behymer of Creative Catering LLC by Molly adds her advice about following a diet low in the aging chemicals. Molly is a friend of mine and an expert in feeding people. She will help us answer the question "What can I eat on this diet?"

Notes from Molly about Following Dr. Walsh's Diet

I appreciate that I am presenting a lot of information that may be new to you. To help you better understand what we're working with, I will begin by reviewing some of the information provided by Dr. Walsh.

Breakfast

Dr. Walsh mentioned eggs. You can prepare them any way you want them—they don't have to be fried. Feel free to add peppers, onions, or any other vegetables to your eggs; just remember to stay away from mushrooms. In addition to eggs, also consider strips of cooked bacon or sliced ham, though you'll want to watch the amount of MSG in these processed meats.

Snacks

In addition to the snacks mentioned by Dr. Walsh, also consider:

- Vegetables (dipped in hummus), olives, and pickles
- Apples, pears, roasted apples, cherries, watermelon, plums, bananas, and grapes

↳   Apples and/or pears sautéed in butter and sprinkled with a bit of cinnamon or cardamom will help alleviate your sweet tooth

Caution: all the above fruits contain significant fructose and many contain significant amounts of citric or tartaric acids. You can eat these foods but be careful of the amount that you eat. Many versions of hummus contain citric acid (or citrus juices) so you should watch for signs of excess intake including itchiness. However, since hummus is useful as a spread on cauliflower, celery, and other foods, let's look at a recipe that does not contain citrus:

Hummus

2	cucumbers
4 c	garbanzo beans, dry, prepared as described below
1/3 c	olive oil
1/2 c	tahini (sesame seed paste)
2–4	garlic cloves
1/8 tsp	cayenne pepper
1 3/4	tsp salt

Dice cucumbers and place them in a strainer, sprinkle them with salt and let them sweat while preparing the other ingredients. (We do this to remove the water from them so that the hummus is not too thin.)

In a blender or food processer, mix the other ingredients until smooth. If the mixture is too thick you can add more olive oil or water.

Place mixture into a mixing bowl and gently spoon in the salted cucumbers.

Chill and enjoy.

Lunch/Dinner:

Foods to consider for your noon and evening meals can include: chicken, pork, beef, beans (all varieties), peppers, onions, kale, lettuce (all varieties), squash, broccoli, zucchini, asparagus, avocado, cabbage, carrots, celery, cucumbers, eggplant, ginger, mashed/boiled potatoes, and/or frozen cut corn.

It's always best for you to prepare your own food rather than buying processed foods. To help you plan your meals, I have included the following recipes. I have restated some of the recipes presented above, and I also provide other recipes.

Food Notes from Molly:

A List of Some Foods That Contain Citric Acid in Their Natural State.

Citrus fruits. Citric acid is in highest concentration in lemons and limes, which are up to 8% citric acid by weight and are a source of commercial citric acid; the more sour the fruit, the higher the citric acid content.

Berries, with the exception of blueberries, contain some citric acid. It is especially found in strawberries, raspberries, gooseberries, cranberries, red currants, and black currants.

Exotic fruits, such as pineapple and tamarind.

Vegetables such as tomatoes (technically a fruit), cayenne peppers (which are not the same as sweet peppers), and sunchokes.

Wine contains citric acid in combination with tartaric acid.

Because these foods (and beverages) contain citric acid, you should be sure to enjoy them—but do not consume them in any level that activates your symptoms.

Eat Your Vegetables—Especially the Green, Leafy Ones

Almost all vegetables are acceptable on the diet (mushrooms should be avoided, and you should limit your intake of potatoes and tomatoes).

Vegetables can be eaten raw, but for many vegetables cooking helps to increase nutrient availability. On the other hand, greens are more nutritious raw because cooking removes their nutrients.

Leafy greens are also a good source of fiber, folate (derived from the word foliage), magnesium, and vitamin K. You may be surprised to know that kale, mustard greens, and bok choy provide readily absorbable calcium—even more than milk! Plus, for only 33 calories, one cup of kale provides 600 percent of the recommended daily amount of vitamin K, 200 percent of vitamin A, and over 100 percent of vitamin C.

There are many methods to make leafy greens more appetizing: you can sauté them with olive oil or butter and garlic, or bake kale chips. You can add them to a manufactured preparation such as chips, or into a smoothie (but be sure to read the list of ingredients on all of your labels before using them—don't assume all packaged vegetables and crackers are going to be free from the aging chemicals).

Seasonings

All spices can be used in this diet, however, some blended seasonings may contain the chemicals we are trying to avoid, so read the labels. If you are using spices that have been dried or mixed with other spices, make sure to check the label for the aging chemicals—or any possible allergens.

Many spices claim to have healing properties. Turmeric, cumin, curry, rosemary, sage, black pepper, nutmeg, and cinnamon are just some of the spices thought to possess brain-healing properties.

A Final Note from Molly

I hope that this diet will help to reverse the distressing symptoms you suffer and will lead you to good health. If you are threatened by mental deterioration, I hope that this diet refreshes you, brings back your mental acuity, and reverses any deterioration. My wish is that it will truly bring you "back to life."

Chapter 13
Molly's Recommended Recipes

Vegetables

Beans

NUTRITION NOTE: Small red beans are the top antioxidant-containing food, while just 1 cup of lentils contains 18 g of protein and 90 percent of the recommended daily foliate intake.

This is a very basic method for cooking dry beans. Because there are many different varieties of beans, the actual cooking times will vary. However, the technique is the same for almost every type of dry bean.

Rinse the beans. Don't be tempted to skip this step, because beans are generally fairly dirty. Run them under cold water in a colander or sieve until the water runs clear.

Put the clean, dry beans into a pot and fill the pot with enough water to cover them. Don't let your beans dry out in the pot—they will become hard and leathery.

This is your chance to add any flavorings you want. I always cook my beans with at least a bay leaf thrown in. I also love boiling them with onions and whole garlic cloves.

Simmer (never boil) the beans—until they're done. Unfortunately, I can't get much more specific than that. Different varieties of beans cook in different ways, so if you are cooking more than one type of bean it is best (but not necessary) to cook them separately. I usually start with 30 minutes on my timer, and then I taste them. If the beans are still hard or chalky inside, I set the timer for 10 more minutes.

NOTE: The one exception to the "simmer" rule is kidney beans. Raw kidney beans contain the toxin phytohaemagglutinin (it's not lethal by any means, but may cause gastrointestinal discomfort and symptoms similar to food poisoning) and must be boiled for 10 minutes to destroy it. Always boil kidney beans for 10 minutes, then reduce the heat and simmer until they are cooked.

Keep checking the beans at regular intervals until they are tender but still firm. (You don't want them falling apart.) The key word here is "simmer."

Once they have reached your preferred consistency, remove the beans from the heat and drain them.

Season the beans using salt, pepper, and olive oil to taste. You can use other spices and herbs, but you may be surprised at how delicious beans are on their own.

Feel free to add boiled or sautéed veggies to this mixture for extra flavor. You can even add meat and some extra liquid to turn it into a hearty soup.

Asparagus

1 lb	fresh asparagus spears, trimmed
1 tbsp	olive oil
	salt and pepper to taste

Grilled Asparagus

Preheat grill to high heat.

Lightly coat the asparagus spears with olive oil. Season with salt and pepper to taste.

Grill over high heat for 2 to 3 minutes, or to desired tenderness.

Baked Asparagus

Preheat oven to 350°.

Lightly coat the asparagus spears with olive oil and season with salt and pepper to taste.

Arrange asparagus on a cookie sheet greased with olive oil or a pan spray.

Bake for 10 to 15 minutes, or to desired tenderness.

Dr. Walsh's Bean and Veggie Lunch Mix

Preparing the bean and vegetable mixtures Dr. Walsh mentioned above will take some time and effort. To use your time most productively, follow his suggestions and prepare it in large batches and freeze it in plastic freezer bags. As it freezes, remove the bags periodically from the freezer and agitate the mixture to prevent the food from freezing into a block of ice.

Beans (dry black beans, garbanzo beans, soy beans, or other dried beans as desired), prepared as above

1 c	peas
1 c	green beans
1 c	asparagus
1 c	frozen corn
1 c	carrots, chopped
	fresh celery, chopped
	fresh spinach, washed and dried
	olive oil and seasonings to taste

Place all ingredients (except beans) in a pan with water and boil for 5 minutes.

In a large bowl, combine the beans with the vegetables.

If using right away, top with chopped celery, and fresh spinach (which will cook due to the residual heat of the vegetables).

If using from frozen, top with fresh celery and microwave on high for 3 minutes. Add fresh spinach and return to the microwave to cook on high for an additional 30 seconds.

Toss with olive oil and other seasonings (be sure that they do not include the aging food chemicals) for extra flavor.

Caramelized Onions

(A treat to add to your beef, pork, or chicken.)

2	large white onions, peeled and sliced
1/4 c	butter

Melt butter in a large saucepan over medium heat.

Stir in onions.

Reduce heat and simmer, stirring occasionally, until onions are translucent and golden, approximately 1 hour.

Sautéed Vegetables

1 tbsp	olive oil
1 tbsp	butter
3	garlic cloves, finely minced
1	jalapeno pepper, seeds and ribs removed, minced
2	zucchini, halved lengthwise and sliced
1	yellow bell pepper, cut into chunks
1	red bell pepper, cut into chunks
1	shallot, sliced
1/4 tsp	salt

freshly ground black pepper to taste

pinch   paprika

Heat olive oil and butter in a large skillet.

Add garlic and jalapeno and cook until softened, about 5 minutes.

Add zucchini, yellow bell pepper, red bell pepper, and shallot; continue to cook and stir until tender, about 5 minutes more.

Season with salt, black pepper, and paprika.

Poultry

Chicken, turkey, and other fowl, simply prepared, are acceptable on this diet. Drumsticks, thighs, and breasts, can be prepared by baking, microwaving, pressure-cooking, slow cooking and through other simple food preparations. (Be careful that any seasoning you use does not contain aging chemicals, such as refined sugar and MSG.)

Chicken with Artichokes

1 tbsp	olive oil
1 tbsp	butter
4	skinless, boneless chicken breast halves
14 oz	marinated, quartered artichoke hearts, drained, liquid reserved
1 c	white wine
1 tbsp	capers
	salt and pepper to taste

Season chicken with salt and pepper.

Heat oil and butter in a large skillet over medium heat.

Brown chicken in oil and butter for 5 to 7 minutes per side. Remove from skillet, and set aside.

Place artichoke hearts in the skillet, and sauté until brown.

Return chicken to skillet, and put in reserved artichoke liquid and wine. Reduce heat to low, and simmer for about 10 to 15 minutes, until chicken is no longer pink and juices run clear.

Stir in capers, and simmer for another 5 minutes, remove from heat. Serve immediately.

Tuscan Chicken

I lb	chicken breast tenders
I/4 tsp	salt
I/4 tsp	black pepper
I tbsp	olive oil
I 1/3 c	onion, sliced
I c	green bell pepper, cut in strips
I tsp	garlic, minced
2 c	chickpeas (precooked)
I/4 tsp	basil
I/4 tsp	oregano
	fresh flat-leaf parsley leaves (optional)

Sprinkle chicken with salt and pepper.

Heat oil in a large nonstick skillet over medium-high heat.

Add chicken to pan; cook 2 minutes on each side or until browned.

Add onion and bell pepper; sauté 4 minutes. Reduce heat to medium.

Add garlic, chickpeas, basil, and oregano. Cover and cook 8 minutes or until thoroughly heated through.

Garnish with parsley leaves, if desired.

Serve immediately.

Rosemary Chicken

I/4 c	butter, melted
I/8 c	olive oil
I tbsp	rosemary
I tbsp	garlic, chopped
	salt and pepper to taste
4	boneless, skinless chicken breasts

Preheat oven to 350 degrees.

In a large bowl or shallow baking pan, combine melted butter, olive oil, rosemary, garlic, salt, and pepper.

Dip chicken into mixture and lay onto a parchment paper-lined baking sheet greased with olive oil or pan spray.

Bake at 350° for 25–30 minutes or until internal temperature reaches 165°.

Serve immediately.

Meat

Beef, pork, and other meats, simply prepared, are acceptable as part of this diet. Meals can include hamburgers, pork chops, and other simply prepared foods (as long as you are careful of the seasoning).

Meat Patties with Egg

1/4 c	chopped carrots
1/4 c	chopped peppers
1	large onion, chopped
1 tbsp	garlic, minced
1 lb	ground beef
1 lb	ground pork
1 lb	ground turkey or chicken
4	large eggs
1/2 c	water
	salt, pepper, and crushed red pepper to taste
1/4 c	chopped fresh parsley (optional)
1/4 c	olive oil (optional)

Coat a large sauté pan with olive oil, add the carrots, peppers, and onion and bring to a medium-high heat. Season generously with salt and cook for about 5 to 7 minutes. (The onion should be very soft and aromatic, but have no color.)

Add the garlic and the crushed red pepper and sauté for another 1 to 2 minutes. Turn off heat and allow to cool. (If you want to skip this step that's okay—you can move on with the warm vegetables.)

In a large bowl, combine the meats and eggs (and optional parsley). It works well to squish the mixture with your hands.

Add the vegetable mixture to the meat mixture. Season generously with salt and squish some more.

Add the water and do one final really good squish. The mixture should be quite wet.

(Test the seasoning of the mix by making a mini hamburger-size patty and cooking it. The mixture should taste really good! If it doesn't, it is probably missing salt. Add more, as needed.)

Preheat the oven to 400° F.

Shape the meat into patties about the size of a flattened tennis ball. Place them on a cookie sheet and bake them in the preheated oven for 30–40 minutes, or until the meat patties are cooked all the way through, not pink. If possible, test with a meat thermometer, removing meat from heat when the internal temperature reaches 165°.

If you're using them right away, enjoy. If you're not using them right away, freeze them for later use after first wrapping them individually in food-grade plastic wrap and sealing them in gallon-sized plastic freezer bags.

Beef Tenderloin Filets

4	beef tenderloin filets
2 tbsp	olive oil
4 tbsp	butter
4	bacon slices (optional)
	salt, pepper, granulated garlic to taste

Preheat oven to 425°.

Rub steaks with olive oil. Season with salt, pepper, and garlic.

Wrap one slice of bacon around the sides of each filet, securing it in place with a toothpick (optional).

Place the filets on a foil-lined baking sheet and top each with 1 tablespoon of butter.

Bake at 425° for 10–20 minutes, or until the filets have reach the desired doneness on a meat thermometer.

Remove from heat and let stand for one or two minutes before serving.

Fish

Tasty fish are also part of our diet. Prepare the fish simply, such as through baking or frying, or try the recipe below.

Pescado a la Veracruzana

2 lb	white-fleshed fish fillets
1 tsp	salt
2 tbsp	oil
1	onion, sliced
2–3	garlic cloves, minced
1 c	water or stock—without aging chemicals
1/3 c	green olives, pitted
3 tbsp	minced parsley
2 tsp	dried oregano
1	bay leaf
1 tbsp	capers, rinsed (optional)
2–3	jalapeño peppers, sliced into rounds (optional)
1	cinnamon stick (optional)
2–3	cloves, whole (optional)
	salt and pepper to taste
	(NOTE: Be careful how much salt you add, because the olives and capers will add their own salt to the sauce and it is easy to overdo it. Because of this, when you make the sauce you will want to wait until the sauce has simmered for a while to taste it before you season it.)

Add the fish and 1 teaspoon of salt to a large bowl and marinate for 30 minutes to an hour.

While the fish is marinating, heat the oil over a medium flame in a large skillet. Add the onions and sauté until they are translucent. Add minced garlic and continue sautéing for another minute.

Add the remaining ingredients—except for the fish. Reduce heat to low and simmer for 10 to 15 minutes to meld flavors and reduce the sauce somewhat. Season to taste with salt and pepper.

Add the fish fillets and cover them with some of the sauce. Reduce heat to low, cover and simmer until fish is cooked through, about 8 to 12 minutes.

Remove from heat and serve immediately.

Pan-Seared Salmon with Dill Butter

2	6-ounce salmon filets
1/2 tbsp	olive oil
2 tbsp	salted butter, room temperature
1/4 tsp	dried dill
1	garlic clove, grated or finely minced
	salt and pepper to taste

Preheat a medium skillet over medium-high heat.

Salt and pepper the salmon filets.

Prepare dill butter by combining butter with dill and garlic in a small bowl. Stir to combine. Set aside.

In the preheated skillet, add the olive oil and cook the salmon (skin side up if it has skin) for 4–5 minutes on the first side, then flip it and cook another 4–5 minutes. The cook time will depend on the size and thickness of your salmon. You want the inside of the salmon to start to turn opaque and reach 135 degrees on a meat thermometer.

After the salmon is cooked, remove from heat and top each fillet with 1 tablespoon of the dill butter.

Serve immediately, or keep refrigerated in an airtight container for up to 5 days.

Index

About the Author

William E. Walsh, MD graduated from Creighton Medical School in Omaha, Nebraska, and served two years in the United States Air Force, where he discovered his fascination with treating allergic diseases. After four years of fellowship at the Mayo Clinic, he passed the examination of the American Board of Allergy and Immunology, which certified him as a specialist in the diagnosis and treatment of allergic diseases. He is also a fellow of the American College of Allergy, Asthma and Immunology.

Following his retirement, Dr. Walsh continues to pursue medical research and to review what he learned in his medical practice. This has led him to a startling conclusion: diet is a major cause of the mental deterioration that causes Alzheimer's disease and other diseases related to damaged and destroyed nerves. He also discovered that he was experiencing early Alzheimer's disease and that he knew how to reverse it.

With this book, he shares this knowledge with you.